INTRODUCTION

THE ROAD TO THE WHITE HOUSE

Each of the 52 presidential elections since 1789 reflects the changing political and social milieu of the United States. Since the second half of the 20th century, presidential elections have also shown the dynamic impact of technology, particularly television. This medium's entrance into the political landscape has changed the way Americans elect their presidents. This book is intended as a guide to the presidential campaigns and election results since the emergence of television.

Television networks began limited coverage of presidential elections in 1948, but the first president to speak to a television camera was Franklin D. Roosevelt in 1939. At that time, radio was the primary mass medium for political communication—one this president was good at using. However, Roosevelt's presidency was the last during which radio was the dominant political medium. His successor, Harry S. Truman, bridged the end of radio's widespread use and the emergence of the age of television.

The Road to the White House Since Television begins with the presidential election of 1948 and ends with the election of 1992. Few would have predicted the results of either election, and it is that unpredictability that makes the subject so interesting and worthy of study.

Each chapter is devoted to a presidential election and is divided into six sections as follows:

1) Setting the Stage: Each election cycle has its distinct flavor, influenced by events taking place in the United States and in the world at the time. This section identifies the political, economic, social and cultural atmosphere of a particular election cycle.

2) The Candidates and the Issues: Short biographies of those candidates receiving over one million popular votes appear in order, from the top vote-getter down. Only in the elections of 1948, 1968, 1972, 1980 and 1992 have third-party and independent candidates reached this one-million-vote figure.

To provide a "political biography," some of the campaign issues and the positions taken by each candidate are merged into this section. Issues were extracted from an examination of party platforms and campaign speeches of individual candidates. Not every issue important to the campaign is included, but the positions emphasized by the candidates are listed.

3) The Campaign: This section identifies some of the highlights and the turning points of the caucus and primary seasons, the conventions and through the individual campaigns up to Election Day.

4) Television and the Campaign: The influence of televised election coverage has increased since television's modest presence in 1948. This discussion attempts to connect television to how presidents get elected.

5) The Results: The election results are reported and put in a historical context. Electoral maps specific to each election year are included.

6) The Postscript: Some of what the elected president did upon assuming the office is mentioned along with excerpted selections from the inaugural address.

"Observing the Rules of the Road," the final chapter, summarizes the changes in the political process seen in the presidential campaigns from 1948 to 1992, and offers suggestions for observing the election of 1996. Essential supporting information and an extensive "Note on Sources" arranged by topic are found in the appendix.

=== 1 ===

THE ELECTION OF 1948

*Population of the United States: **146.63 million***
*Number of eligible voters: **95.57 million***
*Percent of those eligible who voted in 1948: **51.1**; in 1944: **56***
*Percent of television saturation in U.S. households: **0.4***

SETTING THE STAGE

President Harry S. Truman was the incumbent as the 1948 election cycle began. At the 1944 Democratic National Convention, Truman, then a United States senator from Missouri, replaced Henry A. Wallace as the vice-presidential candidate on the Roosevelt ticket. Franklin D. Roosevelt went on to win the 1944 election—an unprecedented fourth term—and Truman, the "Man from Missouri," was positioned next in line to be president of the United States. When Roosevelt died on April 12, 1945, just three months into his new term, Truman assumed the presidency. He came to that office little aware of the awesome decisions awaiting him.

Until Truman occupied the Oval Office, he had scant knowledge of the development of the atomic bomb and thus had to comprehend the weapon's destructive power and potential in a short time. As the World War II conflict was ending in Europe, fighting still raged in the Pacific and the number of American casualties continued to rise. On August 6, 1945, as Truman had ordered, the United States dropped the atomic bomb on Hiroshima, Japan. Three days later a second atomic bomb was dropped on Nagasaki. Within a week, Emperor Hirohito announced Japan's unconditional surrender. The use of the bomb ushered in the Atomic Age and changed the world forever.

Although Truman had brought World War II to a conclusion, he was not a popular president, even among Democratic groups. Parts of the New Deal continued under his administration, but Truman was seen by New Dealers as an interloper or a bland alternative to Roosevelt. Further, Truman's strong support for civil rights in the military and in federal agencies alienated traditionally loyal Southern Democrats.

Truman's lack of support among the Democratic coalition portended bad news for the next presidential election. The Republicans, on the other hand, were optimistic after the 1946 congressional victories that gave them control of both houses of Congress. They had added 11 members in the Senate for a 51 seat to 45 seat majority, and 55 members in the House for a 246 seat to 188 seat majority. After 16 years on the outside, Republicans sensed that moving into the White House in 1948 was a real possibility.

A Gallup Poll taken in October 1948 predicted the Republican presidential candidate, New York Governor Thomas E. Dewey, would win by a landslide. Professional odds-makers made Dewey the prohibitive favorite at 15 to 1. Representative Clare Boothe Luce, a Republican from Connecticut, stated, "Truman is a gone goose." On October 15, the *New York Daily News* remarked, "President Truman appears to be the only American who doesn't think Thomas E. Dewey is going to be elected." And commentator Drew Pearson opined as late as November 1, "Truman put up a courageous fight....But with Dixiecrats and Wallacites against him, he cannot possibly win."

The most audacious pollster, perhaps, was Elmo Roper, who stopped polling on September 9, announcing that Dewey was "almost as good as elected" and that "no amount of electioneering" could elect Truman. As the campaign proceeded, Roper said he detected no reason to revise the edge of 10 to 15 points he had given Dewey. "I stand by my prediction. Dewey is in."

Truman was not without personal resources, however. Known for his vigor and his "can-do" attitude, Truman was able to enliven a war-weary nation when he succeeded the obviously-ill Roosevelt. Many Americans welcomed his common-sense approach to achieving a prosperous peacetime economy. Still, a May 1948 Gallup Poll showed only 36 percent of those sampled approved of the way the president was doing his job. Dismissing the polls, Truman called them "sleeping polls" designed to lull voters into sleeping on Election Day.

As the year 1948 dawned, American industry was at its most productive and Americans had more jobs and higher incomes. The major threat to prosperity was inflation, resulting in part from a series of labor strikes. In July 1948, Truman called Congress back into a two-week special session to consider legislation for his economic and social programs. The legislators did not follow his prescriptions for controlling inflation and improving living conditions. This allowed Truman to blame the Republicans for blocking his plans to better the lot of ordinary Americans.

Further, the American people were unusually perplexed about the international scene this election year. The end of the war was supposed to be a complete victory for world democracy. Yet in April 1948, President Truman launched the $13 billion Marshall Plan designed to prevent the spread of communism by helping rebuild the economies of war-torn countries in Western Europe. The public also thought the country had vanquished its enemies in World War II, but now the United States faced Joseph Stalin in Europe and Mao Tse-tung in Asia. To make matters worse, the threat of a World War III arose when the Soviet Union blockaded the Allied sector of Berlin in June 1948, effectively barring any entry into West Berlin by land. Under Truman's leadership, the Western Allies once again went to Germany. The quickly arranged "airlift" by Allied planes provided food, coal and other supplies to the West Berliners, which eventually led to the lifting of the siege in May 1949. Bernard Baruch, U.S. delegate to the U.N. Atomic Energy Commission, dubbed this confrontational relationship—

between the United States and its Western allies and the Soviet Union and its allies—the "Cold War."

The Candidates and the Issues

President Harry S. Truman, *the Democratic Party candidate*

Truman was born on May 8, 1884, in Lamar, Missouri, a town of about 800 people. On June 28, 1919, he married Elizabeth "Bess" Virginia Wallace, and they lived in her birthplace home in Independence. The couple had one daughter, Mary Margaret.

During World War I, Harry Truman served as a major in the Army. Later he would say that his experience as an officer showed him that he could be a leader. Shortly after the war, Truman and a partner opened the "Truman and Jacobsen" haberdashery in Kansas City and he was soon known as "Haberdasher Harry." The men's apparel store went bankrupt in 1922.

Despite not having an undergraduate degree, Truman attended the Kansas City School of Law. In 1922 he was elected judge of the Jackson County Court in Missouri and became the presiding judge of the same court in 1926. He served until 1934 when, with the backing of the Pendergast political machine, he was elected to the U.S. Senate. In his 1940 re-election bid, he was challenged in the Democratic primary by Governor Lloyd Stark. Stark had the support of President Roosevelt, but Truman, a tough campaigner, defeated the governor and went on to keep his Senate seat.

In 1944, Truman became the U.S. vice president, assuming the presidency in 1945 upon President Roosevelt's death. He served without a vice president until his next term in 1949.

Harry S. Truman died on December 26, 1972, and is buried at Independence, Missouri, on the grounds of the Truman Memorial Library and Museum.

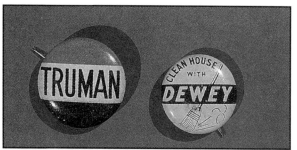

(Campaign materials courtesy private collection of Dr. John Sullivan,
University of Virginia/Photo by Paul Kennedy.)

NEW YORK GOVERNOR THOMAS E. DEWEY,
THE REPUBLICAN PARTY CANDIDATE

Dewey was born on March 24, 1902, in Owosso, Michigan. He graduated from the University of Michigan in 1923 and from the Columbia University law school in 1925. He served in New York as a U.S. attorney from 1932 to 1933, a special prosecutor investigating organized crime from 1935 to 1937 and as district attorney for New York County from 1937 to 1938.

In 1940, Dewey was proposed for the Republican presidential nomination, but he lost out to the eventual nominee, Wendell H. Willkie of Indiana. In that election year, Dewey's first book, *The Case Against the New Deal*, was published.

Elected governor of New York in 1942, Dewey stayed in that office from 1943 to 1955. In 1944 he was also the Republican nominee for president, but lost the general election to Roosevelt.

Thomas E. Dewey died on March 16, 1971.

SOUTH CAROLINA GOVERNOR J. STROM THURMOND,
THE STATES' RIGHTS PARTY CANDIDATE

Thurmond was born in Edgefield, South Carolina, on December 5, 1902. He graduated from Clemson University in South Carolina in 1923. He taught high school from 1923 to 1929 and was a superintendent of education for Edgefield County from 1929 to 1933.

Thurmond studied law on his own and did not attend law school. He was admitted to the South Carolina bar in 1930. From 1930 to 1938, he was a city and county attorney, and from 1933 to 1938 he served in the South Carolina Senate. In 1938 he was appointed a circuit court judge, a post he held until 1942.

During World War II, Thurmond served in the Army in both Europe and the Pacific. In 1946, he was elected governor of South Carolina and remained in office until 1951. He was first elected to the U.S. Senate in 1954 and continues to serve four decades later.

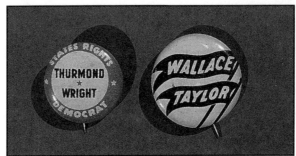

FORMER VICE PRESIDENT HENRY A. WALLACE, THE PROGRESSIVE PARTY CANDIDATE

Wallace was born October 7, 1888, in Adair County, Iowa. He graduated from Iowa State College in 1910 and became the editor of his family's magazine, *Wallace's Farmer*. In 1933, Wallace was named Secretary of Agriculture by President Roosevelt.

In 1940, the Democrats nominated Wallace for vice president. After the Democratic victory, he served as Roosevelt's vice president during World War II from 1941 to 1945. In the 1944 election, he was replaced on the ticket by Harry Truman.

Wallace became Truman's Secretary of Commerce in 1945 and resigned the next year in a dispute with the president over American policy toward the Soviet Union. He then became the editor of the *New Republic* magazine from 1946 to 1947. He broke from the Democratic Party to run as a Progressive in 1948.

Henry A. Wallace died on November 18, 1965.

THE ISSUES

Early in the Cold War, there was a general consensus in the government regarding America's approach to international relations. The accepted policy was to contain the hegemony of the Soviet Union. Republicans and Democrats agreed that international affairs were too important for partisan squabbles, and any debates over policy occurred behind the scenes.Domestic affairs, however, provided fertile ground for political discord.

HARRY S. TRUMAN, DEMOCRAT

President Truman ran a campaign against the 80th Congress. He criticized the Republican majority for preventing the passage of his legislative programs, which he claimed would have rectified some serious economic problems. Truman, proposing a "Fair Deal" that he believed would provide economic opportunity and social equality, campaigned for expanding Social Security, increasing the minimum hourly wage from 40 cents to 75 cents, raising price supports for farmers, expanding affordable housing programs, augmenting aid to education and implementing a national health insurance system. He favored civil rights and called for reducing the national debt. He also demanded the repeal of the 1947 Taft-Hartley Labor-Management Relations Act, which had so irritated labor unions. The act weakened labor's bargaining power by banning "closed shops," which required union membership for employment, and by mandating an 80-day cooling-off period before a strike could occur.

In international affairs, Truman wanted to reduce trade barriers among nations. He advocated increased efforts in containing the spread of communism and a strengthened United Nations to help. He also favored international arms control. In the campaign, he reiterated his support for U.S. recognition of the new state of Israel.

THOMAS E. DEWEY, REPUBLICAN

Dewey charged the Truman administration with corruption. He blamed the Democrats for high taxes, inflated prices and inefficient government.

Dewey favored the expansion of civil rights and was against "racial and religious discrimination" of any kind. He supported the extension of Social Security benefits, maintenance price supports for farmers, employment opportunities for young people, the renewal of urban areas, and he called for assistance for affordable housing. He wanted to reduce the national debt and the inflation rate.

Calling for "a just and lasting peace in the world," Dewey wanted to install international arms controls and to harness the "possibilities of atomic energy." He supported U.S. recognition of the state of Israel.

STROM THURMOND, STATES' RIGHTS

Thurmond split from the Democratic Party at the 1948 convention over its civil rights plank. Claiming his opponents were out to "destroy the American system of balanced power," Thurmond called for states' rights and protested the encroachment of the federal government into state affairs. He advocated local control of police, employment, education and housing. Thurmond opposed the Democrats' Fair Employment Act and favored segregation as traditionally practiced in the South—a separation of the races "where it is considered needful."

HENRY A. WALLACE, PROGRESSIVE

Wallace echoed some of the populist views of earlier progressive candidates, such as William Jennings Bryan, Robert M. LaFollette and James B. Weaver. He opposed the control of the economy by "big business," advocating instead a system of "progressive capitalism." He supported civil rights for all Americans, fair wages for workers and protection for the rights of working people. Wallace called for repeal of the Taft-Hartley Act. He also sought price supports for farmers and lower housing prices for all Americans.

Wallace split with the Democrats primarily on how to approach international affairs. He favored improved relations with the Soviet Union and other communist countries and wanted to seek arms reduction. Wallace believed the United Nations should supervise international assistance. He challenged the rationale and efficacy of the Marshall Plan and criticized the Truman Doctrine—which provided money to Greece and Turkey for defense against any communist encroachment—as being intrusive and unworkable.

THE CAMPAIGN

The election of 1948 provided voters with the usual political symbols and paraphernalia: the Republican elephant; the Democratic donkey and a plentiful supply of whistles; the stars and bars of the Confederate flag for the States' Rights Party; flags with the peace dove and the songs of Pete Seeger and Woody Guthrie for the Progressives. With four major candidates in the race, this was a campaign for political aficionados.

REPUBLICAN NATIONAL CONVENTION,
PHILADELPHIA, PENNSYLVANIA, JUNE 21 TO JUNE 25
In 1948, national conventions still determined the party's nominee, but the quadrennial events were on their way to becoming less important. Candidates and voters were showing more interest in the primaries. Therefore,when former Minnesota Governor Harold Stassen won the Wisconsin and Nebraska primaries, front-runner Thomas Dewey took notice. New Yorker Dewey then won the primary in his neighboring state of New Jersey, but Stassen won in Pennsylvania. Not until the Oregon primary, in a head-to-head battle with Stassen that included Oregon-wide radio debates, did Dewey satisfy Republicans of his vote-getting potential. Dewey's victory in Oregon gave him a clear shot at the nomination and the statewide debates were heard by some party regulars beyond Oregon's borders.

The Republicans nominated Dewey for president and California Governor Earl Warren to be his running mate. For the first time, the party had renominated a previously defeated presidential candidate. The more conservative Republicans settled on Dewey instead of their own favorite, Ohio Senator Robert Taft, because party regulars believed the more moderate Dewey would offend the fewest voters. Tired of losing presidential elections, they were willing to compromise on a sure thing. Though Dewey had lost to Roosevelt in 1944, he now faced Truman, a weaker candidate. Republicans believed that Dewey needed only to stay close to home and away from controversy to bring the party a victory.

Democratic National Convention, Philadelphia, Pennsylvania, July 12 to July 15

Although Truman's popularity was low in the spring of 1948, he did not face a serious challenge in the primaries as his opponent did. There was a move at one point to draft General Dwight Eisenhower to lead the ticket, and even word that Truman might agree to the replacement. Backers wanted the general to run as a Democrat with someone like James Roosevelt, the son of Franklin and Eleanor, as his vice president. General Douglas MacArthur was also floated as a possible candidate. However, both generals declined and would later join the Republicans. Some New Dealers still wanted the former vice president, Henry Wallace. But when the convention settled, it nominated the incumbent Truman for president and Senate Minority Leader Alben W. Barkley of Kentucky, the convention keynote speaker, for vice president.

In the campaign Truman not only faced a unified Republican Party and a moderate candidate, he was challenged within his own party from both the right and the left. Having fought for civil rights measures like integration of the armed forces and nondiscrimination in federal housing, Truman insisted on a strong civil rights plank in the Democratic Party platform. Though Truman's domestic initiatives were generally supported, his actions on civil rights led to the withdrawal of 35 Southern delegates from the convention. The 1948 Democratic convention was tumultuous. Even though delegate walkouts were expected, the impact of the actual occurrence in full view of the press and a budding television audience was stunning.

Truman appeared unmoved by it all and focused on what he saw as the real opponent. "Senator Barkley and I will win this election and make these Republicans like it, don't you forget that," he said in his acceptance speech in Philadelphia. "We will do that because they are wrong and we are right and I will prove it to you." The bravado, however, did not eliminate the political difficulties he faced within his own party.

STATES' RIGHTS DEMOCRATIC PARTY CONVENTION, MONTGOMERY, ALABAMA, JULY 17

The Dixiecrats left the Democratic convention in a dispute over civil rights issues and refused to support Truman or the Democratic Party. They convened two days after the Democrats adjourned. Delegates from 13 states nominated South Carolina Governor Strom Thurmond for president and Mississippi Governor Fielding Wright to be his running mate. By adding another candidate to the field, the sectional party hoped to send the election into the House of Representatives, where they might affect the final result. They thought that, through bartering, they could weaken Truman's commitment to civil rights, or if that effort did not succeed, then prevent his election altogether.

Progressive Party convention,
Philadelphia, Pennsylvania, July 24 to July 25
Disenchanted Democrats, citing their discontent with international affairs and their belief that Truman had not gone far enough on domestic issues, mounted a campaign under the Progressive Party label. Their convention organized the Party and nominated Henry A. Wallace, a former vice president under Franklin Roosevelt, and Idaho Senator Glen Taylor as their candidates. The new party was more a hybrid including some independent voters than it was a complete break from the Democrats. The Progressive candidates and their supporters campaigned vigorously but, in the absence of a party infrastructure, could only take votes from Truman and the Democrats.

Most pundits and pollsters agreed that Dewey would win the election. Republican strategists counseled Dewey not to say anything that might alienate even a small bloc of voters and to stay above the political fray. Dewey wrote his own speeches and ignored Truman as much as he could. In the days before extensive television coverage, this was easy as opposing candidates seldom crossed paths.

Truman, for his part, was willing to fight. The Republicans were eroding his image as a sitting president with well-circulated quips: "To err is Truman" and "I wonder what Truman would do if he were alive?" The president knew that to win he had to answer the challenges and take the offensive from the beginning.

Dewey's train, boldly named "Victory Special," carried him 9,000 miles as he made 100 speeches. Confident that no one could outwork him, Truman knew he could best those numbers. Truman's 17-car campaign train, the "Presidential Special," pulled former President Roosevelt's "Ferdinand Magellan" in the caboose position. The 285,000-ton, bullet-proof train car had been used by Roosevelt during the war and became Truman's platform for speeches to the crowds gathered near the tracks at his frequent "whistle stops." Before television coverage, public appearances by candidates were crucial. Trying to be seen by as many voters as possible and to shake all the hands that could be reached, Truman gave over 350 formal speeches and 250 extemporaneous ones in 36 states. He traveled over 31,000 miles before Election Day. Truman had been campaigning unofficially since June, but Dewey did not venture out onto the campaign trail until September 19, and then did so speaking from his basic text, with only minor variations, each time.

On Labor Day, at the start of his formal campaign, Truman came out of his corner and gave a rousing pro-labor speech to an enthusiastic crowd in Detroit's Cadillac Square. From there his schedule was more like the railroad schedules of the day—not always on time. His campaign appearances were not managed as efficiently as his opponent's, but the crowds responded more spontaneously and robustly.

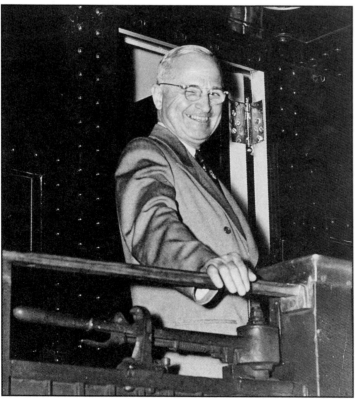

Harry S. Truman traveled over 31,000 miles in his campaign train, the "Presidential Special," and gave over 350 formal speeches. *(Courtesy Library of Congress.)*

Unlike Dewey, who was an accomplished platform speaker, Truman was much better "off the cuff." He spoke directly to the interests of his audiences. He spoke to farmers in straightforward language about their concerns. He mended relations with labor by explaining he would fight for fair wages and against Taft-Hartley. He invited voters to meet his family—his wife, Bess, and daughter, Margaret, whom he called "the Boss" and "the Boss's Boss." Bess and Margaret would simply say "Hello," and the crowd's response showed they identified with the Truman family. Bands greeting Truman would strike up "I'm Just Wild About Harry" and the "Missouri Waltz."

Clark Clifford, special counsel to Truman, spoke for the president's political strategists when he recommended that Truman campaign against the 80th Congress. Truman seemed to relish doing so. Calling it the "do-nothing" Congress and the "worst in history," the president blamed the legislators for stalling his proposals for civil rights, preventing the expansion of Social Security, opposing health insurance for all Americans, blocking fair housing opportunities and holding up his proposals to contain the cost of living. From the back of his campaign train, Truman's voice projected to the back of the crowd: "If you send another Republican Congressman to Washington, you're a bigger bunch of suckers than I think you are." The crowds yelled, "Give 'em hell, Harry!" He called the Republicans "bloodsuckers with offices on Wall Street, princes of privilege, plunderers." And after he got warmed up, he said they were "Wall Street reactionaries" and "gluttons of privilege" who were using the "tapeworm of big business."

Truman made it clear where he stood. He pointed to his achievements: He had taken care of the farmers, protected labor, recognized the state of Israel, furthered civil rights and safeguarded the national interests from Soviet expansion.

As he campaigned, much of the New Deal coalition jumped onto the Truman train—farmers, urban dwellers, blacks, Southerners still loyal to the party, liberals and organized labor. The labor group was particularly important to Truman, who had forced labor to back down from some strikes and weakened their usual vigorous support for

Democratic candidates. This may have cost the Democrats control of Congress in the 1946 mid-term elections. Sobered under a Republican Congress, Truman spoke to labor's needs and told them that they would be much better off under a Truman administration. After Congress passed the Taft-Hartley law over Truman's veto, labor believed him.

In an October 5 letter to his sister Mary Jane, Truman wrote, "It will be the greatest campaign any President ever made. Win, lose, or draw, people will know where I stand and a full record will be made for future action by the Democratic Party."

TELEVISION AND THE 1948 CAMPAIGN

In the summer of 1948, there were fewer than half a million television sets in the country, but by the end of that year the number had doubled. Television network programming was in its infancy, but an established system of radio networks provided a structure upon which to build. The American Broadcasting Company (ABC), the Columbia Broadcasting System (CBS) and the National Broadcasting Company (NBC) were ready to incorporate television into their already existing network structure.

Television cameras captured a political convention for the first time with limited coverage of the 1948 Republican National Convention in Philadelphia. The Republican convention at the end of June was telecast live, accessible only to viewers residing within the reach of big-city signals between Boston and Washington, D.C. At a time when viewers were being attracted by entertainment programs like "Arthur Godfrey's Talent Scouts," "Candid Camera" and "The Milton Berle Show," such information programming was an experiment. Would people stay tuned long enough to watch the politicians finish their speeches?

By today's standards, television technology at the Republican and Democratic conventions was primitive. The broadcast was in black and white and transmission interference provided plenty of "snow."

Unless homes had good antennas, the picture could be unclear and distorted. Further, camera operators on unstable platforms had trouble steadying their cameras. The sometimes shaky pictures from poorly lit convention halls yielded inconsistent results.

Campaign workers knew and cared little about television makeup and staging, but they would soon find that, especially under poor lighting, television magnified visual miscues. The Truman camp learned a lesson about the import of media images when they watched their candidate, wearing a white summer suit, fade away against the convention audience as he delivered his acceptance speech. Truman's voice was clear, but his figure lacked any imposing definition on the black-and-white television screen. Political image-makers had been around at least since Andrew Jackson's "old-hickory" stick, and they would soon learn to adapt this new medium to their candidate's advantage. But at the time, campaign staffs were still more concerned with what their candidates were saying and how it was said and paid less attention to how they looked while saying it. The image of a candidate was built on the written and spoken word and newspaper interpretations of those words. Powerful national newspapers could still make or break candidates. And pictures could be posed, exemplified by the dearth of photographs of President Roosevelt in his wheelchair. The use of television in the 1948 campaign seemed to affect few votes.

Movie newsreels showed Truman to be a fast-walking, forward-moving and forceful-speaking president and an active campaigner. In public appearances, he had developed the ability to be intimate with his audience, but it is unclear whether his intense but "folksy" style worked on the television screen. Dewey's cool demeanor was more controlled and presumably more conducive to capture by the immobile cameras of the time.

On October 5, 1948, the Democrats bought television time on Newark, New Jersey's WATV, Channel 13, for Truman to call the people out to vote and prove the "sleeping polls" wrong. In a sense, it was the first paid political television advertisement. Despite a limited role in the election of 1948, television was an emerging medium presenting possibilities and pitfalls for future candidates. Buying television time would increase the cost of campaigns. The ads and television news coverage would change how Americans elected their presidents.

Television would even influence how presidents governed. Indeed, Truman, the first president to appear on television from the Oval Office, believed the medium would ultimately turn politics into show business.

THE RESULTS

The symbol of the Democrats' 1948 election victory has become the photo of a smiling Truman holding up the November 3 *Chicago Daily Tribune*, its headline blaring "Dewey Defeats Truman." Truman defeated Dewey by 4.5 percentage points in the popular tally and by 114 votes in the Electoral College. The president and the Democratic Party also won the 81st Congress back from the Republicans, 54 seats to 42 seats in the Senate and 263 seats to 171 seats in the House. *The Washington Post*, which had predicted a Dewey victory before the election, welcomed Truman back to Washington with a banner on its office building, "Mr. President, we are ready to eat crow whenever you are ready to serve it."

Truman's victory was enough to satisfy him. He told *The Washington Post* that they could feast on chicken together. But he delighted in imitating radio commentator H.V. Kaltenborn's faulty election predictions. Errors in sampling and methodology had miscued the pollsters. In turn, the political pundits and commentators who had relied on the polls filled the airwaves, newspapers and magazines with misleading political indicators. Scientific polling was still in its infancy.

In retrospect, it is understandable why the prognosticators got it so wrong. The three-way split in the Democratic Party had made Truman's election chances look bleak. And, Progressives drew enough votes from Truman in the states of Maryland, Michigan and New York to cost him those electoral votes. Further, Thurmond took Alabama,

1948

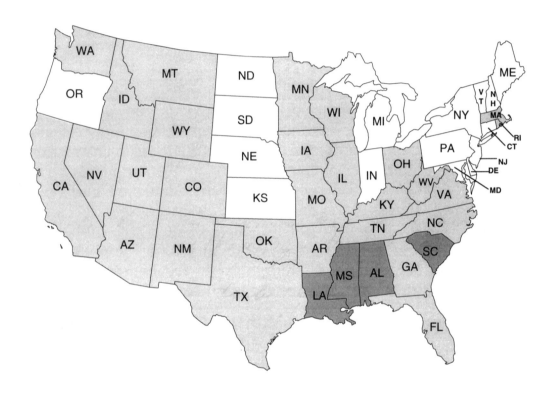

Louisiana, Mississippi and South Carolina, states which had been lodged solidly in the Democratic camp since the Civil War. Yet the "Man from Missouri" won anyway. He had campaigned hard and by retaining much of the "Roosevelt coalition," he was able to frustrate the prognosticators.

◆◆◆

POSTSCRIPT

Harry S. Truman was president for almost two full terms, the first inherited upon the death of his predecessor. By the end of his presidency, he had used his veto 250 times. The Congress overrode 12 of those vetoes.

Truman presided over the dropping of the first atomic bombs, the establishment of the United Nations, the heating of the Cold War, the Berlin Airlift, the launching of the Marshall Plan, the organization of the North Atlantic Treaty Organization (NATO) and the United Nations' "police action" in Korea.

"The American people stand firm in the faith which has inspired this Nation from the beginning. We believe that all men have a right to equal justice under law and equal opportunity to share in the common good. We believe that all men have the right to freedom of thought and expression. We believe that all men are created equal because they are created in the image of God.

From this faith we will not be moved.

The American people desire, and are determined to work for, a world in which all nations and all peoples are free to govern themselves as they see fit and to achieve a decent and satisfying life. Above all else, our people desire, and are determined to work for, peace on earth—a just and lasting peace— based on genuine agreement freely arrived at by equals."

President Harry S. Truman
Inaugural Address
January 20, 1949

= 2 =
THE ELECTION OF 1952

Population of the United States: **157.55 million**
Number of eligible voters: **99.93 million**
Percent of those eligible who voted: **61.6**
Percent of television saturation in U.S. households: **34.2**

SETTING THE STAGE

In the early 1950s, most middle-class men and women still held "traditional" roles in American society—men in the workplace and women in the home caring for the family. In the 1952 election, a new form of political campaigning emerged, the spot advertisement. It specifically targeted women, whose responsibilities made them sensitive to the high cost of living in the inflationary postwar period. Many of these women voters were politically active, meeting to discuss issues and encourage the candidates of their choice.

As the 1952 election approached, Democratic President Harry S. Truman was confronted with international problems. The Chinese Communists, led by Mao Tse-tung, had taken control of mainland China and established the People's Republic of China at Peking on October 1, 1949. The National Chinese government under Chiang Kai-shek was relocated to Taiwan. Communist North Korea invaded the Republic of South Korea on June 25, 1950, and the United States subsequently became entangled in a situation that had the potential of developing into a third world war. With Truman's discharge of General Douglas MacArthur as commander of American troops in Korea in 1951 and continuing news of American casualties in the conflict, the Democratic administration's popularity suffered.

At home, Republican Senator Joseph McCarthy of Wisconsin had been accusing the Democratic Party of being soft on communism. In February 1950, he claimed he had evidence that communists had infiltrated the U.S. State Department. With McCarthy at the helm, the hunt for communists in government continued at a fervent pace throughout the next four years, until the Senate voted in December 1954 to censure McCarthy for his conduct during the period.

On March 30, 1952, Truman announced he would not seek re-election. Pollsters, as they had during the previous election season, declared him to be a persona non grata in politics. In typical Truman style, the president said he vacated the White House with "no regrets." Indeed, in a 1948 diary entry, he had referred to the White House as the "Great White Jail." In 1952 Truman was ready to go back to Missouri with his wife.

THE CANDIDATES AND THE ISSUES

GENERAL DWIGHT DAVID EISENHOWER, THE REPUBLICAN PARTY CANDIDATE

Dwight Eisenhower was born on October 14, 1890, in Denison, Texas, and spent his youth in Abilene, Kansas. On July 1, 1916, he married Mamie Geneva Doud. They had one son who survived past infancy, John Eisenhower.

Eisenhower graduated from the U.S. Military Academy at West Point in 1915, "the class on which the stars fell." Fifty-nine members of his graduating class of 164 became brigadier generals or higher. Eisenhower was awarded a fifth star during World War II after serving as Supreme Allied Commander for the D-Day invasion of June 6, 1944.

In 1948 Eisenhower became president of Columbia University and published his book, *Crusade in Europe*. Some Democrats tried to draft him to replace Truman as their presidential nominee in 1948, but Eisenhower declined and stayed at Columbia. In 1950 President Truman appointed him Supreme Commander of the North Atlantic Treaty Organization (NATO).

Dwight D. Eisenhower died on March 28, 1969, and is buried at the Eisenhower Center in Abilene.

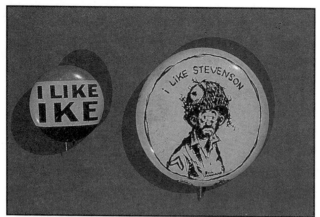

(Campaign materials courtesy private collection of Dr. John Sullivan, University of Virginia/Photo by Paul Kennedy.)

ILLINOIS GOVERNOR ADLAI E. STEVENSON,
THE DEMOCRATIC PARTY CANDIDATE

Stevenson was born on February 5, 1900, in Los Angeles, California. In 1922 he graduated from Princeton University, and in 1926 earned a law degree from Northwestern University. Stevenson practiced law in Chicago until 1933 when he joined the New Deal's Agricultural Adjustment Administration, serving until 1935.

Stevenson returned to government service as a legal advisor to the Secretary of the Navy during World War II. After the war, he was the assistant to the Secretary of State and was involved in the creation of the United Nations in 1945. In 1946, he was a senior advisor to the first American delegation to the United Nations. At age 48, he ran successfully for Illinois governor on a platform to "clean up" the state government. He held that office from 1949 to 1952 and signed 78 "clean-up" laws.

Though Stevenson was from a political family (his grandfather was Grover Cleveland's vice president, 1893 to 1897) he was little known outside the state of Illinois. Stevenson was also divorced, a fact that some thought would prove a hindrance in a national election.

Adlai E. Stevenson died on July 14, 1965.

THE ISSUES

The Republicans summarized their issues in 1952 as the "Seven C's": Change, Control of wages, Cost of inflation, Corea (the old spelling), Communists in government and elsewhere, Corruption in Washington and China's mainland under Communist control.

The Democrats campaigned on American prosperity. Laborers earned good wages, the elderly were more secure due to the expansion of Social Security benefits and teenagers had more summer jobs than ever before. The Democrats adopted the mantra: "You Never Had It So Good." Even so, the American people were in the mood for change. Corruption charges alleged against the powers in Washington involved quid pro quo favors ranging from kitchen appliances to mink coats in exchange for influence on the public policy process. The Democrats also made a political miscalculation in this contest. They campaigned against the "Hoover Depression" even though "Black Thursday," October 24, 1929, was long gone in the minds of the voters.

International affairs, including relations with China, Korea, the Soviet Union and the other communist countries, were on the list of major issues addressed by both parties in the 1952 campaign.

DWIGHT D. "IKE" EISENHOWER, REPUBLICAN

The Republican nominee claimed that five consecutive Democratic administrations had allowed corruption to permeate the power structure in Washington. He blamed the Democrats for the infiltration of communists at home and condemned them for appeasing communism abroad. Eisenhower supported a balanced budget, lower taxes, a reduction in the national debt, a smaller federal government and more fiscal efficiency. He wanted to modify the Social Security system. He also supported the Taft-Hartley Act as a means of reducing labor costs.

The former World War II general pointed to the advantage of having a military man as president during times of international crises. He advocated a stronger national defense and "getting China back" and said he would go to Korea to end the conflict.

ADLAI E. STEVENSON, DEMOCRAT

Stevenson pledged to further the economic prosperity fostered by the past five Democratic administrations and to continue to push the New Deal agenda. He favored expanded civil rights for women, the disabled and other minorities, assistance to poor children and aid for the elderly. Stevenson promised to expand the nation's job base and to increase wages for the average working American. He wanted to repeal the Taft-Hartley Act. He attacked Eisenhower's running mate, Richard Nixon, alleging he had a personal fund provided by wealthy benefactors.

In international relations, Stevenson supported a strong national defense, international disarmament treaties and the Marshall Plan and Truman Doctrine to contain the spread of communism. With regard to Korea, he wanted an honorable peace achieved by maintaining America's "moral position."

THE CAMPAIGN

General Eisenhower had been approached by Democrats to lead their ticket in the 1948 election, but demurred. Early in 1952, he announced that he would be open to a draft from the Republican Party to run for president. "Mr. Republican," Ohio Senator Robert Taft, was in line for the nomination, and he and his supporters had been passed over before. Many Republicans, tired of defeat in presidential elections, believed the conservative Taft could not win, however, and that Eisenhower, thought to be more moderate, would appeal to a broader spectrum of voters.

Eisenhower, the war hero, had no previous Washington record to attack; whereas Senator Taft had a highly visible chronicle of legislative activity and recorded votes including sponsorship of the Taft-Hartley Act. Eisenhower, convinced by Massachusetts Senator Henry Cabot Lodge to enter the New Hampshire primary to test the waters, won the contest. Taft won primaries in Nebraska, Wisconsin and Illinois. Though it was a Taft victory, the Illinois primary was a sign of things to come. Eisenhower, who was not on the ballot, received 147,518 write-in votes and placed third behind Taft and former

Minnesota Governor Harold Stassen. Eisenhower was on the ballot in New Jersey, Pennsylvania and Massachusetts. He won all three and moved closer to the nomination.

President Truman's popularity hovered at around 25 percent in 1952. In March 1952, he announced his decision not to run for another term at a Jefferson-Jackson Day Dinner—traditionally an event at which Democrats celebrate their accomplishments and look toward the future.

THE REPUBLICAN NATIONAL CONVENTION, CHICAGO, ILLINOIS, JULY 7 TO JULY 11

This was the first year for convention floor proceedings to be televised nationally, and Chicago provided a central location for both parties to gather delegates and transmit video signals. Keynote speaker for the Republican convention was General Douglas MacArthur, who received a lengthy ovation when he revealed he had always been a Republican. Enthusiasm ebbed, however, as disputes between Taft and Eisenhower factions over delegate credentials and the "Fair Play" amendment threatened to split the party, much like the Democrats had divided four years earlier. But Senator Everett McKinley Dirksen of Illinois interjected a call for reason in the convention's deliberations by reminding them, "We have had a habit of winning conventions and losing elections in the last 20 years."

The convention named Eisenhower as the Republican presidential candidate and then selected Senator Richard M. Nixon of California to be his running mate. At the convention's end, Eisenhower let Taft know that he could not win without his support. Despite some hard feelings, Taft relented and agreed to endorse his party rival for the presidency.

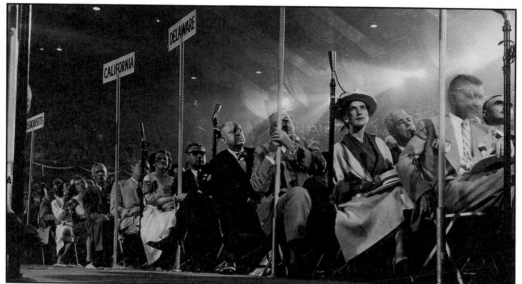

In 1952, the Democratic and Republican conventions were nationally televised for the first time, reaching a viewing audience of over 60 million people. *(Courtesy Library of Congress.)*

THE DEMOCRATIC NATIONAL CONVENTION, CHICAGO, ILLINOIS, JULY 21 TO JULY 26

Preceding the Democratic convention, Senator Estes Kefauver of Tennessee had won most of the Democratic primaries, garnering 64.3 percent of the votes. Regardless of Kefauver's success in the primaries, the results were not binding. Convention delegates wanted a candidate from a large Midwestern industrial state, and party leaders decided on Illinois Governor Adlai Stevenson.

Stevenson had promised the people of Illinois that he would run for a second term as governor and was reluctant to go back on his word. In what would be the last of the multiple-ballot conventions, delegates nominated Stevenson on the third ballot. He finally agreed to lead the ticket on the fourth day of the convention and Alabama Senator John Sparkman was then named to run with him. In his acceptance speech, Adlai Stevenson stated he was "unafraid of ugly truth, contemptuous of lies, half truths, circuses, and demagoguery."

Eisenhower's campaign team beseeched him to adopt a negative tone early on and to avoid the platitudinous neutrality that had plagued the Dewey campaign. Eisenhower urged the "communist-hunters" to find the "pinks" in Washington. He called Washington a "top-to-bottom cesspool." Eisenhower made his negative attacks in generalities, but he permitted Nixon to go after Stevenson personally. With the credibility of a general recently out of combat, Eisenhower bemoaned the "dead and mangled bodies of young Americans" in distant Korean trenches and stated that as president he would forgo the diversions of politics and concentrate on the job of ending the Korean war. "That job requires a personal trip to Korea," he said. "I shall make that trip."

Eisenhower outdistanced Stevenson in train and air travel, with over 50,000 miles covered compared to Stevenson's 32,500. The general gave 228 speeches. Nixon gave 375 speeches and traveled 42,000 miles. Stevenson made 203 speeches and Sparkman made over 400. President Truman campaigned vigorously for the Democratic team and traveled more miles than he had for his own campaign.

Eisenhower's campaign team understood the power of television early. After a difficult primary and convention season in which Taft and Eisenhower had traded charges, the Republicans skillfully projected a unity of the two candidates at the Republican convention. Under the glare of strobe lights, Taft and Eisenhower shook hands for the television cameras in what has come to be known as a "photo opportunity."

One of the most vexing problems that arose in the midst of the campaign was ameliorated through the use of the new medium of television. When Eisenhower's running mate, Richard Nixon, was accused of creating a secret fund of $18,000 to support his personal and political activities, the Republican Party turned to television as a conduit for damage control. Nixon and party leaders concluded that in order to hold onto the nomination, he had to respond publicly to the charges in front of a national audience. Thus, on September 23, 1952, with television time paid for by the Republican National Committee, Nixon gave what became known as his "Checkers" speech. He first

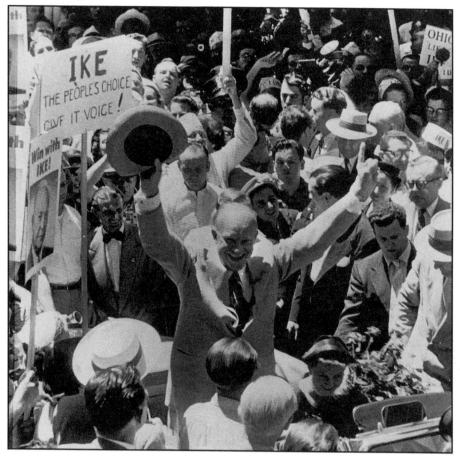

Everywhere he campaigned, Dwight Eisenhower was greeted by supporters carrying "I Like Ike" signs. *(Courtesy Dwight D. Eisenhower Library.)*

laid out his financial history, stressing that he was not rich by the standards of the day. His wife owned a "respectable Republican cloth coat" and not the mink his critics charged. He stood firm on keeping the family dog "Checkers" that the Nixon family had received as a gift. At the end of the 30-minute television appearance, Nixon suggested viewers make their opinions known. Should he resign or continue? Americans sent one million telegrams and letters in support of Nixon to Eisenhower and the Republican National Committee. Moved by the response, Eisenhower announced that Nixon had been "completely vindicated as a man of honor" and kept him on the ticket. Nixon's televised speech may have saved his political career at that time.

Liberal Democrats were enthused about Adlai Stevenson as a candidate. Stevenson was more supportive of civil rights than Truman could afford to be. He wanted to strengthen New Deal programs and vowed repeal of the Taft-Hartley Act. Stevenson also went on the offensive in his campaign, calling Eisenhower's campaign aides, "gutter counselors." Stevenson gave 18 paid televised speeches, each 30 minutes long. These lengthy performances did little to allay the impression some had that he was too intellectual and withdrawn from the public.

Stevenson ran his campaign from Springfield, Illinois, rather than from Washington, putting him close to his duties as governor and to his farm in Libertyville. From there, Stevenson campaigned extensively by airplane, appearing in 32 states. At most of his stops he faced Eisenhower supporters carrying "I like Ike" signs. Meanwhile, the prolonged war in Korea, corruption charges against the Democrats, inflation and the threat of communist infiltration at home and abroad worked against him. These factors, combined with Stevenson's own disdain for canvassing, damaged the campaign.

Television and the 1952 Campaign

The first gavel-to-gavel and nationwide television coverage of the national party conventions occurred in 1952. With over 60 million people watching the conventions this year, stakes were high. Politicians and producers were rushed to find how best to use the new technology to connect with voters.

In this election year, CBS used the UNIVAC computer, which could rapidly report electoral outcomes and immediately update projections based on the vote counts tallied by the new, more accurate technology. The days of a postelection gaffe such as the "Dewey Beats Truman" headline were over. Political analysts marveled at their new abilities, and this rapture would last nearly two decades. In the 1970s, when the extensive use of exit polls on Election Day could predict a winner prior to the closing of all polling locations, controversy erupted over the fairness of these early-prediction practices. Critics believed that voters who had not yet been to the polls would be swayed by television news reports of how the candidates were faring in the early morning and afternoon hours.

Even with the CBS computer breakthrough, the technology for election coverage in 1952 was in its nascent stage. Television pictures in black and white were still "snowy" and dependent on proximity to station transmitters and a clear shot between antennas. Immobile cameras, still frequently shaky, focused on the podium for long periods of time without moving.

Requirements of television were beginning to dictate some of the convention arrangements. Both parties had chosen Chicago for their conventions in part because its central location was a good television transmission point between East and West. In order to have better lighting, the parties agreed to meet in smaller halls, even though they could not accommodate the number of delegates and others who wanted seats. In 1948, camera angles of the speakers were shot from the side; but in 1952, convention speakers could look directly into the camera and at the television audience. Instead of commercial interruptions of the proceedings, a superimposed message like "Philco Brings You the Complete Convention Coverage," periodically appeared on the screen. Although the print press was allowed in to report on the contentious credentials battles in committees at the Republican convention, television cameras were still considered an intrusion and were kept away from the more-telling discord.

By the early 1950s, television was affecting politics in other ways too. It was eroding the influence of political parties. Prior to campaigning via television, electioneering was more direct, hand-to-hand, party-oriented and party-dependent. As the new mediator of campaigns, television afforded candidates a means to reach voters directly rather than through party leaders.

The 1952 campaign was also the first time candidates used advertising firms to shepherd a campaign. The advertising teams for both Eisenhower and Stevenson turned to the new showroom, television. Since television time was more expensive than traditional print and radio media, campaign finance directors became more valued. During this election cycle, the amount of funds raised became closely correlated with the appeal of a candidate or of a party's platform to potential contributors. The financial backers of presidential campaigns began to have a stronger voice in policy formation and campaign strategy.

◆◆◆

THE RESULTS

Eisenhower was the first general to assume the presidency since Benjamin Harrison in 1888. He won 39 states on November 4, giving him 442 electoral votes. He won 55 percent of the popular vote, 33,936,234 ballots. Stevenson won nine states, 89 electoral votes and 27,314,992 popular votes, 44 percent of the final tally. It was "Ike in a landslide." Together, Eisenhower and Stevenson attracted more popular votes than any two previous candidates—over 61 million.

In addition to winning the presidency, Republicans gained control of the 83rd Congress, after having lost the 81st and the 82nd to the Democrats. The House now had 221 Republican seats and 213 Democratic seats. In the Senate, the Republicans narrowly edged the Democrats, 48 seats to 47 seats.

Eisenhower's personal popularity carried the election. He received several million more votes than all Republican congressional candidates together. The landslide victory provided another surprise for the pundits; Eisenhower had cracked the previously solid Democratic South and started the movement toward a two-party South.

Eisenhower's win was his party's first national victory since Herbert Hoover won in 1928. He would probably have won without television, but his campaign staff's ability to use it aided the effort.

1952

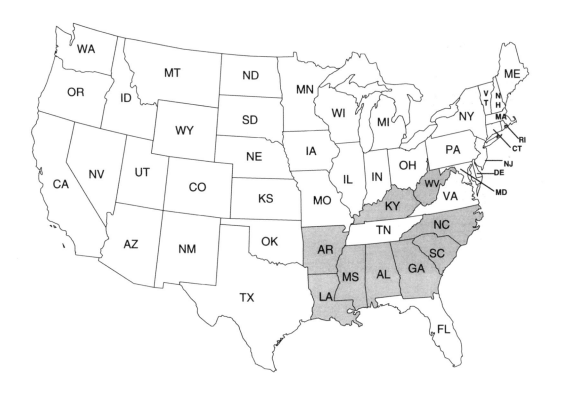

☐ Eisenhower (Republican)

▨ Stevenson (Democrat)

Postscript

Dwight Eisenhower's inauguration was watched on television by Americans from coast to coast. Carried by the Voice of America through kinescopes, it was also seen as far away as Holland and Japan by a worldwide audience estimated at 75 million.

President-elect Eisenhower flew to Korea in December 1952, in his initial effort to "bring the boys home" as he had promised during the campaign. By the summer of 1953, the beginning steps in the withdrawal process were underway. An armistice was signed on July 17, 1953, at Panmunjon, Korea.

In his first term Eisenhower established the Department of Health, Education and Welfare; launched America's first atomic submarine, the *Nautilus*; supported the start of the South East Asia Treaty Organization (SEATO); signed the Communist Control Act of 1954, and approved changes to the Internal Revenue Service Code. Eisenhower was in office when the U.S. Supreme Court handed down the 1954 decision in *Brown v. Board of Education*.

"We know, beyond this, that we are linked to all free peoples not merely by a noble idea but by a simple need. No free people can for long cling to any privilege or enjoy any safety in economic solitude. For all our own material might, even we need markets in the world for the surpluses of our farms and our factories. Equally, we need for these same farms and factories vital materials, and products of distant lands. This basic law of interdependence, so manifest in the commerce of peace, applies with thousand-fold intensity in the event of war.

So we are persuaded by necessity and by belief that the strength of all free people lies in unity; their danger, in discord.

To produce this unity, to meet the challenge of our time, destiny has laid upon our country the responsibility of the free world's leadership.

So it is proper that we assure our friends once again that, in the discharge of this responsibility, we Americans know and we observe the difference between world leadership and imperialism; between firmness and truculence; between a thoughtfully calculated goal and spasmodic reaction to the stimulus of emergencies.

We wish our friends the world over to know this above all: we face the threat—not with dread and confusion—but with confidence and conviction."

President Dwight D. Eisenhower
Inaugural Address
January 20, 1953

= 3 =
THE ELECTION OF 1956

Population of the United States: **168.9 million**
Number of eligible voters: **104.52 million**
Percent of those eligible who voted: **59.3**
Percent of television saturation in U.S. households: **71.8**

SETTING THE STAGE

In the mid-1950s, the average American with access to a television set was watching it for five to six hours a day. Like many American couples at that time, Dwight and Mamie Eisenhower placed their TV trays in front of the television set to watch the top-rated show, "I Love Lucy." In Dwight Eisenhower, the Republicans had the image of a model family man. The president's arresting grin and frequent golf outings placed him in the American mainstream and Mamie's open and familiar presence endeared her to the public. They were appealing as the nation's first family.

Adlai Stevenson's divorce contrasted with the public image of Eisenhower's ideal family life. The fact of his divorce did not play a large role in the 1952 campaign, but as the 1956 election approached, more voters asked whether a divorced man, who conceivably could not handle his own affairs, could handle the country's affairs.

All appeared to be going well for the Republicans until Eisenhower suffered a heart attack on September 24, 1955, while in Denver. The administration's "Operation Candor" quickly reported that his survival was assured, but the public wondered whether Eisenhower would have the stamina to run for re-election. Questions about his health continued when Eisenhower had abdominal surgery in the summer of 1956, the election year.

After the imbroglio in Korea ended with the truce in July 1953, the nation turned its attention to a complex domestic scene. On May 17, 1954, the U.S. Supreme Court ruled in *Brown v. Board of Education*, striking down the notion of "separate but equal" and declaring segregated schools unconstitutional. In a second decision, May 31, 1955, called *Brown II*, the Court ordered schools desegregated "with all deliberate speed." This mandate would have an impact on Eisenhower's second term, and his response would have far-reaching implications for subsequent administrations.

The movement to desegregate education continued to meet resistance even after the *Brown* decisions. In January 1956, the Alabama State Senate passed a resolution nullifying *Brown*. In February, Virginia's legislature adopted a resolution challenging the Supreme Court's desegregation order and asserting the right of the state to interpose its sovereignty: The state of Virginia would allow public moneys to be used to fund private schools, thereby bypassing compliance with the *Brown* decisions. In March, 101 senators and representatives from Southern states requested their states to resist desegregation "by all lawful means."

Americans could now watch the unfolding of world events on television, and international affairs continued to draw their attention. In October 1956, Israel occupied the Sinai Peninsula and Great Britain and France took the Suez Canal from Egypt. Also in October, the Hungarian revolt against Russian dominance and their own Communist government was suppressed by the Soviets at a cost of thousands of Hungarian lives. Toward the end of the year, December 2, Fidel Castro landed in Oriente Province on his mission to overthrow Cuban leader, Fulgencio Batista.

The nation was comfortable with Eisenhower and the economic situation, and he enjoyed residual good will from those who credited him with ending the Korean conflict. With international crises looming, the prospect of a military man continuing to hold the office of president was reassuring to many Americans.

The Candidates and the Issues

The 1956 presidential tickets for the Republicans and the Democrats were almost the same as in 1952; only the Democrats' nominee for vice president differed. Once again it was Eisenhower, now the incumbent president, versus Stevenson, the former Illinois governor. Their biographies appear in chapter two.

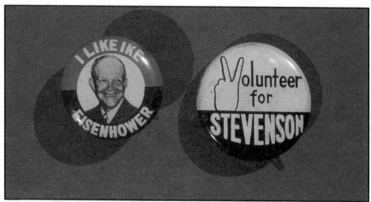

(Campaign materials courtesy private collection of Dr. John Sullivan, University of Virginia/Photo by Paul Kennedy.)

The renominated Adlai Stevenson left the choice of his running mate to the delegates in an unusual open convention. Their choice, Tennessee Senator Estes Kefauver, was known as an organized-crime fighter, a reputation boosted in the early 1950s when his Senate hearings on organized crime and racketeering were televised nationally. He won the nomination after overcoming a challenge by the young senator from Massachusetts, John F. Kennedy.

The Democrats had done something else unconventional. A losing Democratic candidate had not been renominated to run against the same person who defeated him in the previous election since William Jennings Bryan ran against William McKinley in 1896 and again in 1900.

THE ISSUES

The American people, looking for stability during international crises and enjoying a general prosperity, were not inclined to change leaders. Even though some farmers were unhappy about the level of price supports they received and laborers thought they were paid too little, the country was in a mood for moderation and Eisenhower fit the political milieu to a tee.

Some voters had concerns about things the candidates at this juncture had little control over: Eisenhower's health, Richard Nixon's reputation and Stevenson's divorce. None of these issues surfaced as political fodder for the campaign, but they were touched on in the media and in living rooms across the land. Personal issues were not yet material for public exposure and exploitation.

DWIGHT D. EISENHOWER, REPUBLICAN

Looking to sustain the strong economy, Eisenhower proposed a balanced budget and lower taxes. He favored the relationship between federal and state governments mandated by the Constitution. A supporter of the Taft-Hartley Act, he advocated collective bargaining between labor and management without government interference. He stood for further elimination of discrimination in the military and government.

The president could point to his leadership experience and to the country's peace and prosperity during his administration. He supported maintaining U.S. strength abroad and would continue the peacetime draft and proceed with above-ground nuclear testing. In international relations, he urged "mutual economic and military cooperation among the free nations, sufficient to deter or repel aggression wherever it may threaten."

ADLAI E. STEVENSON, DEMOCRAT

Stevenson continued his emphasis on social welfare and environmental issues, looking to abolish poverty and reduce pollution. He pledged to support small businesses, agricultural programs and price supports and the use of nuclear power for peaceful purposes. He wanted to repeal the Taft-Hartley Act and end the peacetime draft. The former governor favored civil rights for everyone, fair and full employment opportunities and the desegregation of schools, as directed by *Brown II*, with "all deliberate speed."

Stevenson also accused the Republicans of practicing "graft and corruption" and dispensing special privileges. His criticism of Vice President Richard Nixon reminded the voters of the possibility that Nixon could become president.

Pointing out errors in Eisenhower's handling of international relations, Stevenson favored reliance on the United Nations for most international problems. He supported worldwide disarmament, the halt of above-ground nuclear testing in hopes of reducing pollution and a moratorium on the testing of H-bombs.

◆◆◆

THE CAMPAIGN

The candidates' use of television in this contest allowed them to reach many more people than they had in 1952. There would be no Dewey-like campaigning for either of them.

In February, Eisenhower declared he would run again in spite of his heart attack. Coached and cued by actor Robert Montgomery, the president announced his decision to run to 65 million television viewers. Apparently in good health, the president won the New Hampshire primary and every other primary he entered and was in effect unchallenged going into the convention.

By 1956, the primaries had become a factor in determining the presidential nominees. The early spotlight provided by television coverage could spur or hinder a campaign. After Kefauver won the New Hampshire primary on the second Tuesday in March and then took Minnesota, it became clear that Stevenson needed to come out and engage him if he wanted the nomination. Stevenson defeated Kefauver in several hard-fought primaries. By the time the Democratic National Convention began, Kefauver had won

New Hampshire, Minnesota, Wisconsin, New Jersey, Maryland, Indiana, Nebraska, Montana and South Dakota; and Stevenson had won his home state of Illinois, Alaska, Pennsylvania, Oregon, Florida and California. Though the convention delegates would still make the final decision, Stevenson's primary victories in the big delegate states gave him the delegate lead going into the Democratic convention.

THE DEMOCRATIC NATIONAL CONVENTION, CHICAGO, ILLINOIS, AUGUST 13 TO AUGUST 17

The Democrats had something of a contest on their hands. Tennessee Senator Estes Kefauver challenged Stevenson for the nomination. Kefauver, the tall, Yale-educated, border-state senator in his coonskin cap, cut an imposing figure and was popular among the rank and file. Stevenson had two other challengers—New York Governor Averell Harriman and Senate Majority Leader Lyndon Johnson from Texas. Eleanor Roosevelt endorsed Stevenson, but former President Harry Truman came out for Harriman. "My fight is against the Republicans," Stevenson responded to his challengers, "not against any Democrat."

The Democrats returned Adlai Stevenson to the top of the ticket, this time on the first ballot. Stevenson then said, "I have decided that the selection of the vice-presidential nominee should be made through the free processes of the convention." Delegates of the "open" convention chose Estes Kefauver over Massachusetts Senator John F. Kennedy. During the up and down balloting, the television audience was introduced to the Kennedy family as they followed the contest and tallied the voice votes.

THE REPUBLICAN NATIONAL CONVENTION,
SAN FRANCISCO, CALIFORNIA, AUGUST 20 TO AUGUST 23
With improved television lighting and the camera's tendency to add weight, the effects of Eisenhower's illnesses were not apparent to the millions of convention viewers at home. Former Minnesota Governor Harold Stassen tried to "dump" Nixon from the ticket, but the Republicans wanted to keep their winning team. When the tenacious Nixon was nominated along with Eisenhower at the Cow Palace, all hands were on board.

◆◆◆

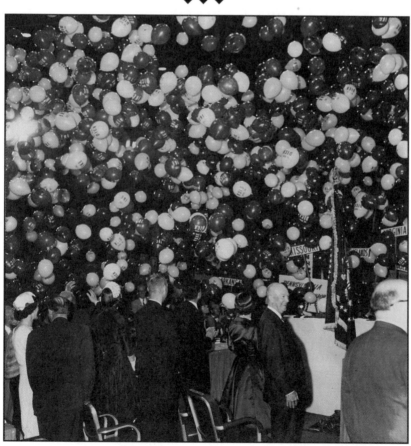

Red, white and blue balloons were let loose at the Republican National Convention as President Eisenhower was renominated to contest challenger Adlai Stevenson for a second time. *(Courtesy Library of Congress.)*

Labor Day once again signaled the start of the presidential campaign. Truman had popularized the modern whistle-stop campaign and Eisenhower's team made good use of the "bandwagon." This oversized float carried cameras, microphones, a plentiful supply of the traditional campaign materials: bunting, buttons, brochures and bumper stickers, and red, white and blue balloons. In each community visited by the "Ike Wagon," the band played and the "Ike girls" cheered.

Television allowed Eisenhower to campaign in all 48 states without extensive personal travel. Still recovering his health, Eisenhower made full use of this opportunity. The president still traveled 14,000 miles and visited 13 states. Eisenhower's personal physician, Dr. Howard McCrum Snyder, had pronounced him fit to run, saying with at least a twinge of resignation that the president "would prefer to die with his boots on."

Stevenson moved his campaign headquarters from Springfield, Illinois, to Washington, D.C. In an attempt to communicate better, he adjusted his manner of speaking and some of his policies and worked at becoming more of a talker and less of an orator. He shook more hands and listened to more people. The Democratic team out-traveled the incumbent, going three times as many miles. On these trips, Estes Kefauver wore his trademark coonskin hat and Adlai Stevenson wore his shoe with a hole in the sole, a familiar symbol from an ad in the previous campaign. Stevenson and Kefauver meant these appearances to convey that they were not elitists, but rather imbued in the Democratic tradition Andrew Jackson had started—the common man as candidate.

Roles reversed in 1956. In the presidential elections of 1936 through 1952, Republicans were on the outside mounting the attack. Now that they were in office, they were in the unaccustomed but enviable position of defending an incumbency. They adapted well.

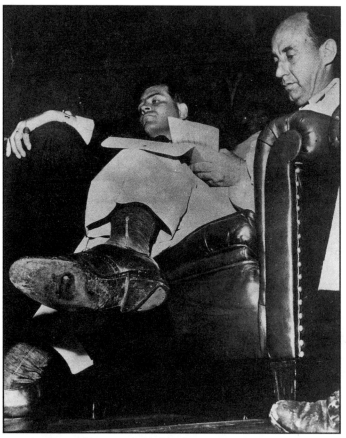

Adlai Stevenson continued to wear his trademark shoe with a hole in the sole and campaigned as "the common man." *(Courtesy of Smithsonian Institution.)*

TELEVISION AND THE 1956 CAMPAIGN

By 1956, politicians and pundits realized that television mattered. They were just not sure how much. More certain of the power of television campaigning over personal appearances was Hugh Scott, the Republican national chairman. "Most will not hear what he says," said Scott about the candidate. "What's that to getting into every voter's living room?" Some have speculated that before television Eisenhower's health may have prevented him from running, but Eisenhower's campaign team was able to construct an effective television campaign. Democrat Stevenson, who generally disliked campaigning, was willing to do more this time. His extensive travel schedule was pitted against Eisenhower's use of television.

At the conventions, in addition to scores of technicians who connected the television cables that crisscrossed and circulated the convention floor, the networks employed commentators, reporters, political pundits and celebrities. John Daly led the ABC reporting team, Walter Cronkite and Robert Trout headed CBS newscasters, and David Brinkley and Chet Huntley anchored for NBC. Television's black-and-white images were much sharper this year, and pictures from portable cameras that followed the candidates from the holding rooms to the convention platform added a sense of drama even when there may have been none. Realizing that network cameras could capture their foibles as well as their triumphs and relay both to their constituents, the political parties emphasized good behavior.

For the first time, campaign spending on television advertising outstripped what was spent on radio. With only three television networks, advertisers could saturate the airwaves and reach most viewers. To help pay advertising costs, Democrats sold a $25 campaign booklet, "TV for Victory Fund—Keep Stevenson and Kefauver on TV." For their part, the Republicans presented Eisenhower as the leader of peace and prosperity and placed their commercials in a time when most people were watching.

Just under 35 million homes had television sets, accounting for about two-thirds of all homes and about double the number in the previous campaign, just four years earlier. The commercial and political opportunities which came with the growing prevalence of television changed the way campaigns were conducted. Both major parties were aware of the numbers this new medium could attract and scheduled their activities around the times they could reach the most viewers. Republicans were especially aware of the increased voting power of women and targeted some of their televised events and ads to this demographic group. Television was about to make a difference in the election process, but it would take another election for that to happen.

THE RESULTS

"U.S.A. Likes Ike." The headline of the *Boston Daily Globe* on November 7, 1956, noted a landslide victory for the president. At age 66, Eisenhower was now the oldest incumbent president to be re-elected and the first Republican president to win re-election since William McKinley in 1900. He was also the first elected president since Zachary Taylor in 1848 to have virtually no electoral coattails; the Republican congressional candidates failed to win a majority in either chamber. The Democrats gained both houses of Congress. They now held a 49 seat to 47 seat edge in the Senate, and a 234 seat to 201 seat edge in the House of Representatives.

Women reportedly voted in large numbers for Eisenhower. When asked why, they typically said they feared a war and wanted the stable family man with a military background in the White House.

In the general election, Stevenson won several states in the traditionally Democratic South but he lost almost everything else including his home state of Illinois. President Eisenhower made inroads into the broader Democratic South. Eisenhower added Louisiana, Oklahoma and Texas to Florida, Tennessee and Virginia, which he had also won in 1952. At 1:45 the morning after his landslide, Eisenhower made his victory statement, calling for the Republican Party to move beyond criticism of the New Deal and toward application of traditional Republican principles to contemporary problems, a "Modern Republicanism."

1956

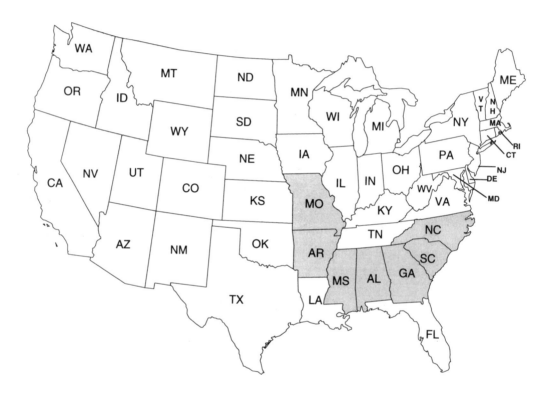

Eisenhower (Republican)

Stevenson (Democrat)

POSTSCRIPT

President Eisenhower issued the Eisenhower doctrine, January 5, 1957, which stated the willingness of the United States to defend against communist infiltration in the Middle East. In July 1958, the president acted on the pledge, sending troops to Lebanon to help put down the disorder there. The Soviet Union's *Sputnik I* went into space on October 4, 1957. In response, Eisenhower signed the National Defense Education Act of 1958, intended to use the school curriculum to bolster America's defense system. In June 1956, he executed the Federal Aid Highway Act authorizing a national highway system. The president signed the Civil Rights Act of 1957, establishing the Civil Rights Commission and a division for civil rights enforcement in the Department of Justice. On September 25, 1957, the president sent the 101st Airborne into Little Rock to hold back those who wanted to prevent the integration of Central High School. In 1960, Eisenhower endorsed provisions that were added to the Civil Rights Act, strengthening its voting rights sections.

When Dwight Eisenhower entered his first term as president, there were 48 stars in the flag of the United States; when he left office, Alaska and Hawaii had been admitted to the union and the American flag had 50 stars. President Eisenhower presided over two terms of general prosperity, interrupted by two brief recessions. By the end of his second term, the number of people on Social Security had doubled, and he had spent more on public works than his predecessors in his effort to modernize America. He was relieved that after extricating U.S. troops from Korea in 1953, his two terms were war-free.

Eisenhower kept a plaque on his desk in the Oval Office, *"Su Avitar in Modor, Fortiter in Re,"* a Latin phrase meaning "Gently in Manner, Strongly in Deed."

"We honor, no less in this divided world than in a less tormented time, the people of Russia. We do not dread, rather do we welcome, their demands for more intellectual freedom, greater security in their demands for more intellectual freedom, greater security before their own laws, fuller enjoyment of the rewards of their own toil. For as such things come to pass the more certain will be the coming of that day when our people may freely meet in friendship.

So we voice our hope and our belief that we can help to heal this divided world. Thus may the nations cease to live in trembling before the menace of force. Thus may the weight of fear and the weight of arms be taken from the burdened shoulders of mankind.

This, nothing less, is the labor to which we are called and our strength dedicated.

And so the prayer of our people carries far beyond our own frontiers, to the wide world of our duty and our destiny.

May the light of freedom, coming to all darkened lands, flame brightly— until at last the darkness is no more.

May the turbulence of our age yield to a true time of peace, when men and nations shall share a life that honors the dignity of each, the brotherhood of all."

President Dwight D. Eisenhower
Second Inaugural Address
January 20, 1957

— 4 —
THE ELECTION OF 1960

*Population of the United States: **180.67 million***
*Number of eligible voters: **109.67 million***
*Percent of those eligible who voted: **62.8***
*Percent of television saturation in U.S. households: **87.1***

SETTING THE STAGE

According to the 1960 Census, about 70 percent of the people in the United States lived in urban areas, a fact that made urban issues more important in this election year than they had been before. Other demographic changes since the 1950 Census revealed a changing social fabric in America. For example, the number of women participating in the work force continued to grow. And more than 2.5 million new immigrants came to the United States.

In 1960 the inflation rate in the country stood at 1.7 percent and unemployment was at 5.5 percent. In his final State of the Union address to Congress, January 7, 1960, President Eisenhower projected a $200 million budget surplus for the year. All economic indicators were not positive, however. American farmers' criticism of price supports and a residue of the 1958 recession created doubts about the administration's economic programs.

The Cold War with the U.S.S.R. was still going strong. On May 1, 1960, the Soviets shot down an American U-2 reconnaissance plane flying over their airspace and captured the pilot, Francis Gary Powers. After an initial American denial, President Eisenhower admitted on May 7 that the plane was on a spying mission. This did nothing to thaw relations with the Soviets. Soviet leader Nikita Khrushchev proceeded to revoke an invitation to Eisenhower to visit the Soviet Union and canceled Soviet participation in the scheduled Paris summit meeting.

At home, the Civil Rights Act of 1960 empowered the federal government to enforce civil rights through Justice Department intervention. Increased civil rights unrest persisted throughout President Eisenhower's second term, and these stirrings portended even greater activity to come during the 1960s. The Republican Party approached the 1960 elections with some apprehension. The party had suffered defeat in the congressional elections of 1958, losing 13 seats in the Senate and 47 seats in the House. In September of 1958, Eisenhower's chief of staff and special assistant, Sherman Adams, resigned because of allegations that he had accepted gifts from lobbyists. The incident embarrassed the Republicans and the president because of their pledge to clear the government of influence peddling. With such a climate and with Eisenhower barred from a third term by the 22nd Amendment, Republican confidence needed a boost.

Vice President Richard Nixon had been an unassuming representative for the president and had stood in for Eisenhower during his recuperation. Nixon had withstood hostile crowds hurling objects and anti-American epithets in South America and had held his own in the now famous "kitchen debate," an encounter with Khrushchev over technology. Nixon could be diplomatic and deferential, but he was also a tough political infighter. In a 1946 congressional race in California, Nixon had suggested that some communists supported his opponent. He won that election. Allegations about the loyalty of his opponent again cropped up in a 1950 Senate race against Helen Gahagan Douglas—Douglas was tagged the "Pink Lady." Richard Nixon won the Senate seat and would remain a part of the American political scene for a long time.

THE CANDIDATES AND THE ISSUES

MASSACHUSETTS SENATOR JOHN FITZGERALD KENNEDY,
THE DEMOCRATIC PARTY CANDIDATE

Kennedy was born on May 29, 1917, at the family home in Brookline, Massachusetts, and spent a lot of time in his youth at the Kennedy summer home in Hyannis Port on Cape Cod. He married Jacqueline Lee Bouvier on September 12, 1953, in Newport, Rhode Island. The couple had one daughter, Caroline, and one surviving son, John Jr.

Kennedy was from a large, politically active family. His father had served as U.S. Ambassador to Great Britain, and his mother's father had been a mayor of Boston. John Kennedy graduated from Harvard in 1940. During World War II from 1941 to 1945, he served in the Navy. In 1946 he was elected to the U.S. House of Representatives from Massachusetts and served until 1953, when he assumed the Senate seat he had won from the incumbent, Henry Cabot Lodge. He served in the Senate from 1953 to 1961. Kennedy was unsuccessful in his attempt to secure the vice-presidential nomination at the 1956 Democratic convention. His book about acts of courage in American politics, *Profiles in Courage*, was awarded the Pulitzer Prize for biography in 1957.

President Kennedy was assassinated on November 22, 1963, and is buried at Arlington National Cemetery.

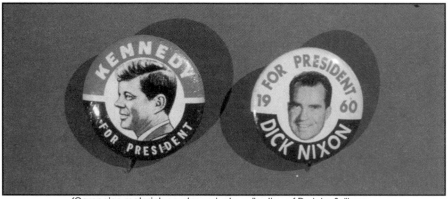

(Campaign materials courtesy private collection of Dr. John Sullivan,
University of Virginia/Photo by Paul Kennedy.)

VICE PRESIDENT RICHARD MILHOUS NIXON,
THE REPUBLICAN PARTY CANDIDATE

Nixon was born January 9, 1913, in Yorba Linda, California. He married Thelma Catherine "Pat" Ryan on June 21, 1940. The couple had two daughters, Patricia and Julie.

Nixon graduated from Whittier College in California in 1934 and from the Duke University law school in 1937. After practicing law for five years, he joined the Navy, serving during World War II, and became a lieutenant commander.

In 1946, he defeated the Democratic incumbent and served two terms in the U.S. House of Representatives from California. In 1950, in part because of his reputation as a fighter against communism made in the Alger Hiss case, he won a seat in the U.S. Senate and served until 1953, when he became vice president of the United States. Nixon held the office during both Eisenhower administrations.

Richard Nixon died on April 22, 1994, and is buried near the Richard Nixon Library in Yorba Linda, California.

THE ISSUES

An underlying issue in this campaign was that Kennedy, if elected, would be the first U.S. president who was a practicing Roman Catholic. Kennedy made a point of saying he supported the "complete separation of church and state." In a political contest between a Quaker, Richard Nixon, and a Catholic, both candidates avoided the issue of religion, but it was a factor for many Americans.

JOHN F. KENNEDY, DEMOCRAT

Kennedy campaigned for a lengthy domestic agenda: higher teacher salaries, more aid to public schools and no federal aid to parochial schools; renewal of urban areas; stronger civil rights legislation; a consumer protection council; health insurance coverage for senior citizens through the Social Security system; more good jobs, and a national Peace Corps that would provide service to other countries.

He favored limits on campaign contributions, advocated protection of the environment and natural resources and wanted to accelerate the space program.

Kennedy vowed to reduce the alleged "missile gap" between the United States and the Soviet Union. He called for more defense spending and international arms reduction. He wanted to provide aid to underdeveloped countries and would support anti-Castro Cubans in their attempt to change Cuba's government.

RICHARD M. NIXON, REPUBLICAN

The vice president called for strengthening civil rights measures, but did not favor busing as a means to achieve school desegregation. He wanted to reduce the national debt. He would extend unemployment benefits, conserve natural resources and develop atomic energy for peaceful purposes. He came out in favor of the line-item veto.

Nixon advocated more defense spending. He opposed the moratorium on nuclear weapons testing, without adequate inspections, and favored the development of defensive weapons. He proposed a strong anti-communist policy in dealing with other nations and called for the exclusion of mainland China from the United Nations.

THE CAMPAIGN

Endowed by his family's fortune, the young Kennedy had money to promote his candidacy. The Massachusetts senator entered seven widely scattered primaries and won each one. Senator Hubert H. Humphrey, his main opposition in the primaries, was discouraged by Kennedy's clean sweep and stopped his active pursuit of the nomination after losing the West Virginia primary. Senate Majority Leader Lyndon B. Johnson of Texas and Missouri Senator Stuart Symington waited for the convention to contest the nomination. By winning the primaries, however, Kennedy showed party leaders and delegates that he was what they looked for, a vote-getter. The primaries, particularly in West Virginia, demonstrated that, if Kennedy made the case that religion would not interfere with his policies, his religion was not an issue.

The choice for the Republican nominee was decided early. New York Governor Nelson Rockefeller looked as if he would make a serious run at Vice President Nixon, but pulled out on December 26, 1959. This left Nixon time to build a campaign. There would be no internecine battles within the Republican Party in 1960. The more conservative Republicans had been beaten in 1958, and those remaining knew moderation was necessary if they were going to win in this election year. Nixon seemed to be the most logical choice. He had served Eisenhower well, was a tough campaigner and had connections with both wings of the party. As a result of this consensus, Nixon had less opposition to divert his attention during the primary season than did his Democratic opponent.

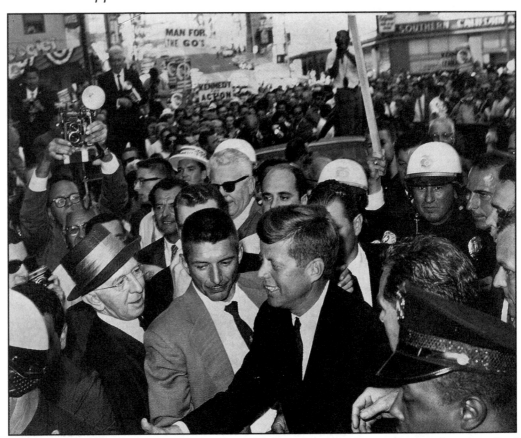

John F. Kennedy, a young senator from Massachusetts, showed party leaders that he was a vote-getter and won the Democratic nomination. *(Credit: Consolidated News Pictures/Photo by G.E. "Gene" Forte.)*

REPUBLICAN NATIONAL CONVENTION,
CHICAGO, ILLINOIS, JULY 25 TO JULY 28

By convention time, only Arizona Senator Barry M. Goldwater was still mentioned by Nixon's opponents as a possible alternative. The balloting for the presidential nomination began with Louisiana. Goldwater received only 10 of that state's 26 votes and promptly withdrew. Vice President Nixon was nominated on the first ballot and Goldwater asked the convention for its full support. Delegates then unanimously selected former ambassador to the United Nations Henry Cabot Lodge of Massachusetts to be the vice-presidential nominee. After Lodge lost his Senate seat to John Kennedy in 1952, he served for seven years as U.N. ambassador. Lodge was the grandson of Senator Henry Cabot Lodge, who had opposed Woodrow Wilson's League of Nations after World War I.

DEMOCRATIC NATIONAL CONVENTION,
LOS ANGELES, CALIFORNIA, AUGUST 24 TO AUGUST 27

Kennedy's winning streak continued. After defeating all comers in the primaries, he agreed to debate Lyndon Johnson before their respective delegations, Massachusetts and Texas, just prior to the convention balloting. It was more a "joint response" than a debate, and Kennedy held his own against the more experienced majority leader. He held up well enough to win on the first ballot at the convention, 806 votes to 409 votes over Johnson. Missouri Governor James T. Blair Jr., who had put Senator Symington's name in nomination, called for the convention to unanimously support Kennedy. The convention did. Kennedy then chose the Southerner he had held back at the convention, Lyndon Johnson, to balance the ticket and placate party insiders. Kennedy and Johnson matched roughly the geographic balance of the

1932 Democratic team, Franklin Roosevelt from New York and John Garner from Texas.

Adlai Stevenson was another possible candidate. Supporters of the two-time nominee were still "Madly for Adlai," but they did not want to chance a Democratic loss. Delegates had been wooed by Kennedy, this new, vigorous and photogenic candidate. To top off the convention, John Kennedy moved the event from the convention hall to the Los Angeles Coliseum to give his "New Frontier" acceptance speech to 80,000 people. Close-up shots of the candidate as he was looking toward a setting sun made dramatic pictures for television viewers.

As the general campaign commenced, Vice President Nixon used his experience holding national office and dealing with Khrushchev against the less-experienced senator. Kennedy cited his 14 years in Congress as a counter to charges that he was too young, at 43, to handle the presidency. Kennedy attacked the "do-nothing" Eisenhower administration, claiming that Republican lassitude had led to a missile gap in the Soviet Union's favor.

Less than two weeks after his Labor Day beginning, Kennedy made his statement on the religion question. Speaking to the Greater Houston Ministerial Association, he said he believed in an impenetrable wall between church and state and if his office required him to either "violate my conscience or violate the national interest" he would resign. "Contrary to common newspaper usage," Kennedy told the ministers, "I am not the Catholic candidate for President. I do not speak for my church on public matters—and the church does not speak for me."

Both candidates supported the effort to improve civil rights in the United States, with little distinction between their two positions. Martin Luther King Sr., father of the civil rights leader, actually supported Nixon early in the campaign. When his son was jailed in Birmingham, Alabama, for protesting against city policies toward blacks, both John Kennedy and his brother Robert called the younger King's family to express concern. This event received a lot of attention in the campaign, helping Kennedy. As Kennedy called for King's release from jail, he won over a large portion of black voters including the elder King, who was known to have political influence among the parishioners in his own church and beyond.

By Election Day, Kennedy had not only the Catholic vote, but the black and the labor voting blocs too. In a close election, this proved crucial.

Nixon knew the Democrats had roughly a 60 percent to 40 percent edge in party registration and campaigned extensively. He was the first candidate to campaign in every state. There were now 50 states including newly admitted Alaska and Hawaii. Nixon gave over 150 speeches, visited 188 cities, traveling 65,000 miles, some in "Dick and Pat Nixon's Campaign Victory Train." John Kennedy went to 44 states, traveling 44,000 miles and making about 120 speeches. Johnson worked the South for the Democratic team and Lodge covered the West and the Northeast for the Republicans.

After securing the nomination, Kennedy challenged Nixon to debate. Nixon's campaign manager recommended against giving the lesser-known opponent a place on the same platform but Nixon, confident in his abilities to debate, accepted. Dates for the televised debates were set: September 26 in Chicago; October 7 in Washington, D.C.; October 13 with Nixon in Hollywood and Kennedy in New York; and October 21 with both candidates in New York. Over 66 million people watched the first debate originating from the studio of station WBBM-TV in Chicago.

TELEVISION AND THE 1960 CAMPAIGN

As television coverage became the focus of political campaigns, the contests played out increasingly in the nation's living rooms. The productions rivaled entertainment shows. Rostrums at the conventions were equipped with elevators so that all speakers would appear on camera at eye level. Speakers wore stage makeup under the bright lights and took advice from actors and media professionals on their performances. Image-makers, now significant players in the campaigns, were thought to be instrumental in the outcome of the first televised presidential debates and the election.

Large television monitors, mounted around the convention halls for the first time, gave those attending a close view of the speakers and a look at the interviews being telecast to the home viewers. Television was having an impact, inside and outside the hall.

The Women's Committee of the Democratic National Committee suggested that women invite a dozen friends to their homes to have "Coffee with Senator and Mrs. Kennedy," a vicarious experience watching the candidate and his wife campaign on television. Both Jacqueline Kennedy and Pat Nixon campaigned more actively than candidates' wives had to that point.

Kennedy's use of campaign ads in 1960 was skillful. Repetition, "Kennedy, Kennedy, Kennedy...," increased his name recognition. Eleanor Roosevelt's appearance in "Citizens for Kennedy" heightened his stature. And footage from his debates with Nixon reinforced the positive impression he had made. In 1952 and 1956, the Republicans had been ahead in using television technology, but in 1960 the Democrats had the edge.

A noteworthy change in this election was the increasing influence of pollsters and campaign advisors who specialized in reading and interpreting public opinion. Kennedy hired pollster Louis Harris, who became one of his inner circle of advisors. The Republicans soon followed suit, hiring their own experts.

Televising of the 1960 presidential debates was possible because of the suspension of the "equal time" provision, Section 315 of the Communication Act of 1934. Section 315 mandated that broadcasters issuing air time to any candidate running for public office must give equal time opportunities to all other candidates for that office. A 1959 amendment exempted newscasts, news interviews, incidental appearances in documentaries and on-the-spot news coverage, but not debates, from compliance with the equal time provision. However, in 1960, a one-time suspension, applying to presidential and vice-presidential candidates, allowed networks to put the two major candidates on stage without giving valuable time to other candidates listed on the ballot. ABC, CBS and NBC provided time for four debates between Kennedy and Nixon. It was the first time the major parties' nominees had appeared on the same stage at the same time and the first time before television cameras.

The 1960 debates were reminiscent of the Lincoln-Douglas debates in the contest for a U.S. Senate seat from Illinois in 1858. But there were big differences. Abraham Lincoln and Stephen A. Douglas had three hours for each of their seven joint appearances. In recent debates, for the highest office in the land, candidates have generally only three to four total hours divided between them and the moderator or reporters. Lincoln and Douglas debated without a moderator or any intervention from the press. Partisan newspapers of the time spun their stories afterward.

Nixon's confidence going into the debates was soon affected by the visual component of television. Television tends to favor vertical lines, hence assisting the taller Kennedy, who also appeared tanned, rested and freshly shaven. Kennedy wore a dark blue suit and light blue shirt in the first debate to contrast with the gray background of black-and-white television. Nixon's gray suit blended into the background and the lighting accentuated his usual slight beard. He had refused more than a touch of makeup for the first debate, but would employ it for the others. Add this to his recent 20-pound weight loss because of illness, the fact that he perspired under the hot lights and rocked back and forth because of a leg ailment, and Nixon had a problem with this primarily visual medium. Kennedy was aware of the red light on the "hot" camera and spoke directly to it. Nixon's less effective eye contact made him seem unsteady and less sincere. The result was that the video presentation of the debates told a different story than the audio version. Reports indicated that radio listeners generally thought Nixon fared better than Kennedy, while those watching television generally gave Kennedy the edge.

The debates, if nothing else, increased Kennedy's drawing power. Crowds surging to meet him provided action for television cameras looking for a story, and the dramatic footage found its way onto the burgeoning nightly news shows. Kennedy's name recognition soon equaled that of the vice president.

As early as the 1960 campaign, some Americans were concerned about style obscuring the substance of the election issues. More and more in the following years, viewers would acclimate to the smooth veneer of "packaging." This packaging has become an issue in itself, with claims that eye-pleasing images can overcome a weak message.

In the end, Kennedy said that it was "TV more than anything that turned the tide." Some political observers believe that the television age of politics started with the 1960 election. Indeed, the Republican nominee for vice president, Henry Cabot Lodge, was chosen in part because as U.N. ambassador he had received considerable television exposure in New York City, an audience considered essential for a Republican victory.

◆◆◆

THE RESULTS

The election of November 8, 1960, was one of the closest in American history and was not official until January of 1961. Kennedy won by less than 0.2 percent of the popular vote. In 1888, Benjamin Harrison actually lost the popular vote by 0.8 percent, but won in the Electoral College. Kennedy edged Nixon by 118,574 popular votes out of a total of nearly 69 million; 49.7 percent of the popular vote to 49.5 percent. Some have estimated the margin to be less than two votes a precinct. Kennedy won more comfortably in the Electoral College, 303 votes to 219 votes for Nixon.

Results showed that Kennedy won the industrial states because he had the backing of most Catholics and attracted the voting blocs of blacks and labor. Nixon did well in some Southern states, in the West and in some farm states. Kennedy took 22 states to Nixon's 26 states.

1960

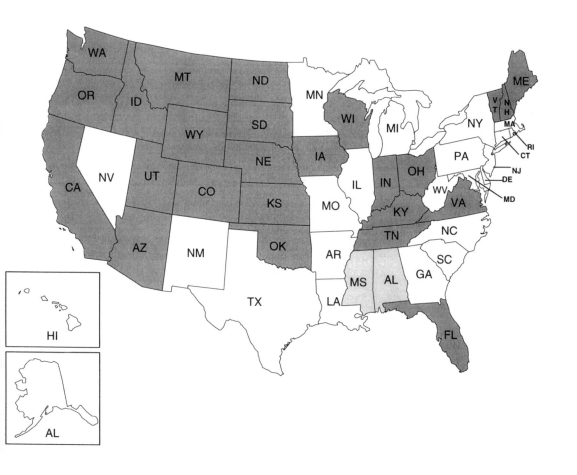

Kennedy (Democrat)

Nixon (Republican)

Byrd (Democrat)

Had Illinois and Texas gone the other way, it would have been Nixon in 1960, but when Illinois joined the Kennedy column, the election in the Electoral College went to the senator from Massachusetts. Most of Alabama's electoral votes and all of Mississippi's went to Senator Harry Byrd of Virginia, who was also on the ballot. The six additional Electoral College votes from the new states of Alaska and Hawaii were split equally, with Alaska's three delegates going for Nixon and Hawaii's three delegates voting for Kennedy.

The Democrats lost some of their strength in Congress but still remained in control. They had a 64-seat to 36-seat advantage in the Senate and, despite a loss of 20 seats in the House, maintained a majority of 263 seats to 174 seats. Many voters were tired of "deadlock" in government and wanted a president and Congress of the same party. They now had it.

POSTSCRIPT

In the two years and 306 days of his administration, Kennedy signed the Alliance for Progress charter in August of 1961, which provided billions of dollars for Latin America; he approved military support for over 1,500 Cuban exiles who invaded their homeland on April 17, 1961, but American support failed to materialize in time to save the invasion. He signed the Manpower Development and Training Act in 1962. Kennedy's "New Frontier" pledge launched the concept of a national Peace Corps serving foreign countries and an active space program. In May 1961 Alan Shepherd become the first American in space and in February 1962 John Glenn became the first American to orbit the Earth.

The Berlin Wall separating East and West Germany went up in 1961, supported by the Soviets. During the Cuban Missile Crisis in October 1962, Kennedy confronted the Soviets and averted a military conflict. He signed the Nuclear Test Ban Treaty with the Soviet Union and Great Britain in July of 1963. President Kennedy was less successful in his efforts for civil rights. He also fell short of his goals in mass transit and medicare legislation.

◆◆◆

"So let us begin anew—remembering on both sides that civility is not a sign of weakness, and sincerity is always subject to proof. Let us never negotiate out of fear. But let us never fear to negotiate.

Let both sides explore what problems unite us instead of belaboring those problems which divide us.

Let both sides, for the first time, formulate serious and precise proposals for the inspection and control of arms—and bring the absolute power to destroy other nations under the absolute control of all nations.

Let both sides seek to invoke the wonders of science instead of its terrors. Together let us explore the stars, conquer the deserts, eradicate disease, tap the ocean depths and encourage the arts and commerce.

Let both sides unite to heed in all corners of the earth the command of Isaiah—to 'undo the heavy burdens ... and to let the oppressed go free.'

And if a beach-head of cooperation may push back the jungle of suspicion, let both sides join in creating a new endeavor, not a new balance of power, but a new world of law, where the strong are just and the weak secure and the peace preserved."

President John F. Kennedy
Inaugural Address
January 20, 1961

= 5 =

THE ELECTION OF 1964

*Population of the United States: **191.89 million***
*Number of eligible voters: **114.09 million***
*Percent of those eligible who voted: **61.9***
*Percent of television saturation in U.S. households: **92.3***

SETTING THE STAGE

After John Kennedy's assassination in Dallas on November 22, 1963, Vice President Lyndon Johnson took the oath of office aboard Air Force One. Probably no one had taken over the presidency with as much knowledge and ability to use the office as Lyndon Baines Johnson. Almost immediately, the former Senate majority leader was able to use his considerable legislative skills to begin converting the thousand days of the Kennedy administration into a thousand pieces of legislation.

On July 2, 1964, Johnson signed the Civil Rights Act of 1964, which prohibited discrimination in voting, jobs and public accommodations. The president had guided the omnibus bill through Congress with the bipartisan assistance of the Senate minority leader, Republican Everett Dirksen of Illinois and the Senate majority whip, Democrat Hubert Humphrey of Minnesota. After the Senate invoked cloture to end 75 days of filibustering, the president had his bill. The purpose of the Civil Rights Act, said Johnson at the televised signing, "is not to divide, but to end divisions." On July 30, Johnson signed the Medicare Act, holding the ceremony in Independence, Missouri, to honor former President Harry Truman, who had advocated such coverage for the elderly in his 1948 campaign. When Johnson signed the Economic Opportunity Act of 1964 in August, he identified it as one Texas-size step in his own broad program for social justice, the "War on Poverty."

Johnson sent more legislation to Congress than any president since the New Deal era, personally guiding much of it through the many stages of the legislative process. He also signed more legislation into law than almost any president before him. Though Johnson had been an active vice president under Kennedy, it was clear from the beginning that his Texas upbringing had not prepared him to play second fiddle. As president, Johnson assumed a more comfortable role in the lead.

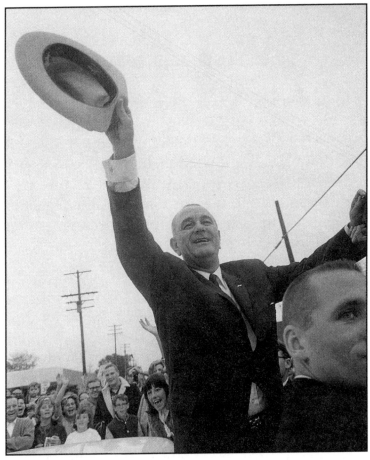

Before assuming the presidency, Lyndon B. Johnson served as a U.S. Representative and a U.S. Senator from Texas, and as vice president under John F. Kennedy. *(Courtesy LBJ Library Collection/Photo by Cecil Stoughton.)*

In response to the reported attack by North Vietnam on two U.S. destroyers on August 2, 1964, Congress passed the Gulf of Tonkin Resolution, giving the president authority to "take all necessary measures to repel any armed attack against forces of the United States and to prevent further aggression" by North Vietnam. In October of the same year, Nikita S. Khrushchev was ousted as premier of the Soviet Union and replaced by Leonid Brezhnev as first secretary of the Communist Central Committee and Aleksei N. Kosygin as premier.

The bodies of three young civil rights workers from Mississippi and New York, who had been missing since June, were found buried near Philadelphia, Mississippi on August 4. The FBI aided the search for those responsible, but convictions proved difficult to obtain. In Atlanta, Georgia, Lester G. Maddox closed his Pickrick Restaurant to avoid a federal order that he serve black patrons. Previously, he had armed his customers with axe handles to prevent the integration of his eatery. On January 10, 1967, Maddox was sworn in as Georgia's governor.

The Warren Commission report, released in September 1964, determined that Lee Harvey Oswald acted alone as President Kennedy's assassin. Oswald had been shot fatally by Jack Ruby while being moved to a safer jail on November 24, 1963. Ruby was convicted of Oswald's murder in March 1964. This year also saw a federal jury convict the president of the International Brotherhood of Teamsters, James R. Hoffa, of jury tampering.

In 1960, New York was still more populous than California by a margin of one million residents, but Americans continued to move west. In 1964, the U.S. Census Bureau reported that California had finally exceeded New York in total population, and in electoral votes. An additional change in the number of electoral votes came with the 1961 ratification of the 23rd Amendment to the Constitution, which enfranchised residents of the District of Columbia in national elections. They voted for a president for the first time in 1964.

THE CANDIDATES AND THE ISSUES

PRESIDENT LYNDON BAINES JOHNSON,
THE DEMOCRATIC PARTY CANDIDATE

Johnson was born on August 27, 1908, at his family's home near the towns of Stonewall and Johnson City, Texas. He spent his boyhood in that area and the latter part of his life at the LBJ Ranch in Stonewall. Johnson married Claudia Alta "Lady Bird" Taylor on November 17, 1934. The couple had two daughters, Lynda and Lucy.

Johnson graduated from Southwest Texas State College in 1930 and taught high school for a year before becoming secretary to a congressman in Washington. He was Texas director of the New Deal's National Youth Administration from 1935 to 1937. During World War II, he served as a lieutenant commander in the Navy.

Elected to the U.S. House of Representatives from Texas in 1936, Johnson served in that body from 1937 to 1949. He won a Senate seat in 1948. In the Senate he was the Democratic whip from 1951 to 1953 and the majority leader from 1953 until 1961 when he became vice president to John F. Kennedy. In 1963 after Kennedy's assassination, Johnson assumed the presidency.

Lyndon Johnson died on January 22, 1973, and is buried near his LBJ Ranch.

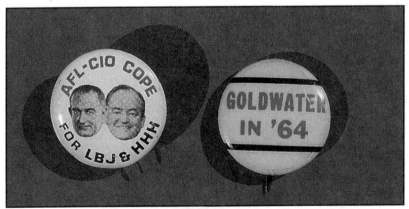

(Campaign materials courtesy private collection of Dr. John Sullivan, University of Virginia/Photo by Paul Kennedy.)

Arizona Senator Barry M. Goldwater, the Republican Party candidate

Goldwater was born January 1, 1909, in Phoenix, Arizona. He went to the Staunton Military Academy and spent a year at the University of Arizona. He went to work at the family's Phoenix department store in 1929 and by 1937 was its president. In World War II, he was a pilot in the Air Transport Command's military branch.

Goldwater ran successfully for the Phoenix City Council beginning his term in 1949. He won a U.S. Senate seat in 1952 and was re-elected in 1958.

Conscience of a Conservative, Goldwater's political and economic credo published in 1960, sold almost as many copies as John F. Kennedy's *Profiles in Courage*. After the 1964 election, Goldwater continued to serve in the Senate before retiring to Arizona in 1983.

◆◆◆

THE ISSUES

In the 1964 election, President Lyndon B. Johnson had the country's peace and prosperity going for him, a tough combination for a challenger to contest. The economy looked strong and American involvement in Vietnam had not yet escalated.

Barry M. Goldwater wanted to reduce government rather than expand it. His hard-line stance on Vietnam and his unwillingness to negotiate with the communists without concessions were perceived by many as threatening an expansion of the conflict. Goldwater sought to provide voters with "a choice not an echo." In Conscience of a Conservative, *Goldwater said that government should ensure and encourage individual freedom and otherwise leave people free to manage their own affairs. He built his candidacy on those principles.*

Lyndon B. Johnson, Democrat

President Johnson sought to build a "Great Society" that ensured medical care for older citizens, a decent income for farmers and an education for every child "to the limit of his ability." He endorsed civil rights and condemned extremism in both the political left and right. He also supported environmental issues.

Johnson pledged to defend freedom in the world and move all nations "toward peace instead of war." He planned to contain the conflict in Vietnam so it would not expand and resisted the use of even low-grade nuclear weapons in the conflict. Johnson wanted to keep the control of nuclear weapons in the hands of the U.S. president.

BARRY M. GOLDWATER, REPUBLICAN

The challenger campaigned against a big federal government and for the repeal of some of the New Deal's social programs. He favored ending federal aid to education, reducing farm subsidies and opposed federal involvement in desegregating schools. Goldwater called for encouraging "a free and competitive economy" while maintaining "a stable monetary and fiscal climate." He sought to reform the tax system and to revise Social Security, proposing a voluntary program rather than a mandated expenditure. Goldwater strongly advocated enforcing law and order, stating that public officials had to keep the streets safe from "bullies and marauders."

Goldwater opposed nuclear test ban treaties and called for construction of a defense system to protect the United States against missile attack. He favored giving NATO commanders authority over the use of tactical nuclear weapons in defense of NATO countries. He called for the ouster of Communist China from the United Nations. On Vietnam, Goldwater wanted to defeat the communists rather than co-exist with them and to bomb North Vietnam to speed the end of the war. He was willing to win battles diplomatically, but supported military solutions if peaceful efforts failed.

THE CAMPAIGN

Lyndon Johnson learned his politics in Texas observing his elders. His father, Sam Ealy Johnson Jr., a former state legislator, and his uncle Clarence Martin were skilled politicians and showed him how to get elected and stay that way. His mother, a former teacher and editor, taught him how to communicate. Unlike some earlier candidates, Johnson saw the usefulness of the new modes of campaigning and adapted to current technology. Though he was not a natural on television in the beginning, he understood what the medium could do and took advantage of it.

After assuming the presidency, Johnson proposed his War on Poverty legislation and other measures and showed what he could do, even with a "conservative" Congress. Although Democrats were in the majority, many of them were from the conservative South. His Civil Rights Act passed in an even stronger version than what Kennedy had proposed. He got an $11.5 billion tax cut, despite its threat to balloon the deficit. In the 1964 election cycle, Johnson tried to bring more of his own kind of New Deal Democrats into Congress.

The leading contenders for the Republican nomination in 1964, with the exception of Senator Barry Goldwater, were all governors, Nelson Rockefeller of New York, George Romney of Michigan and William Scranton of Pennsylvania. Rockefeller appeared to have a good chance but his campaign fizzled when he remarried, reminding the public that he had been divorced, still a political taboo in 1964.

In the primaries, Henry Cabot Lodge of Massachusetts, the candidate for vice president in 1960, won in New Hampshire as a favorite son over Goldwater and Rockefeller. Goldwater went on to win Illinois, Texas, Indiana, Nebraska and California. Rockefeller won Oregon, but Goldwater edged him by a little over 3 percentage points in the crucial state of California.

REPUBLICAN NATIONAL CONVENTION, SAN FRANCISCO, CALIFORNIA, JULY 13 TO JULY 16

Republicans had a more contentious convention than the Democrats. Front-runner Goldwater was challenged on the convention floor by William Scranton and by Senator Margaret Chase Smith from Maine. Scranton even challenged Goldwater to a public debate at the convention but the debate did not happen. Senate Minority Leader Everett Dirksen nominated Goldwater saying, "Could there be a more devoted person to the Constitution than Barry Goldwater, the peddler's grandson?"

Trying to offer an alternative to Goldwater and what he saw as a sure election defeat, Nelson Rockefeller struggled with the convention crowd for enough order to be heard. Goldwater supporters roared disapproval at Rockefeller's defiance, and amid the boos Rockefeller exclaimed, "It's still a free country, ladies and gentlemen."

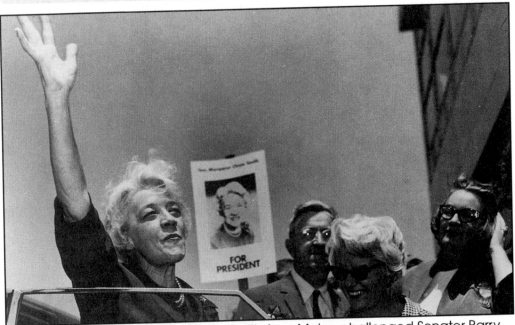

In 1964, Senator Margaret Chase Smith from Maine challenged Senator Barry Goldwater for the Republican presidential nomination.
(Courtesy Smithsonian Institution.)

Senator Barry Goldwater was selected on the first ballot and Representative William E. Miller of New York was named as his running mate. Two sentences from Goldwater's acceptance speech invited headlines the next day: "I would remind you that extremism in the defense of liberty is no vice. And let me remind you that moderation in the pursuit of justice is no virtue."

DEMOCRATIC NATIONAL CONVENTION, ATLANTIC CITY, NEW JERSEY, AUGUST 24 TO AUGUST 27

From the start it was clear that the Democratic convention had Lyndon Johnson's stamp on it. By and large, the American people believed they were prospering and would do even better in the future. Johnson was at the height of his popularity, and no Democrat was about to seriously challenge him.

Despite the Tonkin Gulf incident and resolution, the Vietnam conflict was still viewed as a distant problem. Johnson said that he would not "send American boys nine or 10 thousand miles from home to do what Asian boys ought to be doing for themselves."

The Democratic Party unanimously selected Lyndon B. Johnson as its candidate for president. Not having been elected to the office on his own right, Johnson was not going to take any chances and he was not going to be overshadowed at his own show. In choosing his running mate, he overlooked former Attorney General Robert F. Kennedy for the more predictable Senator Hubert Humphrey of Minnesota. The ticket of Johnson and Humphrey was a formidable one, combining geographical balance with copious political experience.

Johnson campaigned widely, but like other front-runners stayed away from saying anything that could get him into political trouble with any constituency. He stayed for the most part above the fray until September, when he campaigned for 45 days, making over 200 speeches and traveling 60,000 miles, a new record for an incumbent. Johnson was seeking a total victory.

Some Americans perceived Goldwater as "trigger happy" in defense issues. This impression was exploited by the Democrats in the campaign and led to the creation of the so-called "Daisy Girl Ad." The black-and-white television commercial featured the reflection of a nuclear explosion in the eye of a young girl plucking daisy petals, and in the background a countdown and then the voice of Johnson: "These are the stakes....we must either love each other, or we must die." The message "Vote for President Johnson on November 3" flashed on the screen. The television ad was perhaps the most negative political commercial made to this point and many felt the not-so-subtle implication was going too far. The Democrats decided against running it again. The television networks, however, ran clips from the "Daisy Girl" on news programs in the following days.

Late in the campaign, Lady Bird Johnson traveled from Virginia and proceeded into the South in one of the last "whistle-stop" campaigns. It was an important trip at a time that the Democrats' traditional political alliances in the South were threatened by the Civil Rights Act. The "Lady Bird Special" was Harry Truman's idea. "There are still a hell of a lot of people in this country who don't know where the airport is," he told Johnson. "But they damn sure know where the depot is. If you let 'em know you're coming, they'll be down to listen to you." Truman wanted to give the Republicans "hell" one last time.

Goldwater's campaign took him 75,000 miles around the country. In his canvass, he proposed a "Can-Win Foreign Policy." His supporters circulated a "Precinct Education Manual" that stated his positions: "Political power should be wielded forthrightly to dissuade non-communist or nonaligned nations from supporting communism in foreign policy. As in most areas of human relationships, the wisest and most honorable rule of conduct is to reward one's friends and to punish one's enemies. The Democratic administration...stands this rule on its head."

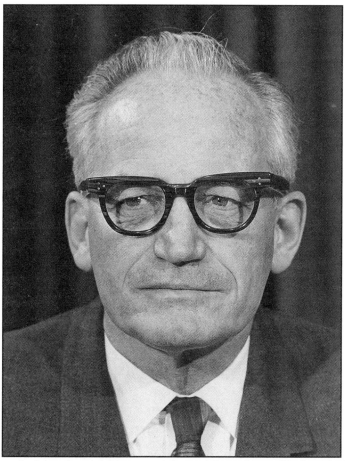

Senator Barry Goldwater said he would provide voters with, "a choice not an echo," and took a hard-line stance on Vietnam. *(Credit: Consolidated News Pictures/Photo by Gene Forte.)*

The Republicans also used negative campaigning and believed they had a lot of ammunition, political and personal, to use against Johnson. A problem for the Republican campaign, however, was Goldwater's own frankness, which frequently got him into trouble with political constituencies he could not afford to alienate. He half-heartedly speculated whether the country would not be better off if the eastern seaboard were sawed-off, and he suggested significant revisions in Social Security, possibly making it voluntary. As the nation's population was getting older, this age group was gaining in voting power and influence. Their voting bloc was more attracted to Johnson's proposals for medical care and expanded Social Security benefits.

TELEVISION AND THE 1964 CAMPAIGN

By 1964, traditional campaign techniques such as parades, whistle-stop speeches at train depots, baby kissing and handshaking at the factory gate were no longer political devices in and of themselves, but were part of the backdrop for events staged for the television cameras.

Conventions especially provided colorful sets for television. Balloons dropped from the ceilings on cheering crowds and gave cameras some of the action they needed to keep an audience's attention. Johnson had learned how to use a teleprompter. Delivering his speech at the Democratic convention, he was able to maintain good eye contact with the television audience. As Johnson said "I accept your nomination," the tight camera shot erased any "visual noise" that would detract from the powerful image.

With multiple contenders for the nomination, the Republican convention provided the most drama. Nelson Rockefeller, challenging the nomination of Goldwater against an unruly audience, created compelling television when he admonished the chair, "You control the audience and I'll take my five minutes."

That the major party conventions were held in different cities increased the networks' costs in carrying them, yet they attracted large audiences, yielding high ratings. A reported 42 million people tuned in at one time or another to the Democratic National Convention. Held in Atlantic City, New Jersey, in one of the largest convention halls on the East coast, the convention was the largest yet, hosting an estimated 6,000 journalists and newscasters. The possibilities of closed-circuit cable transmissions were put on display here for the first time as interviews with public officials were cablecast to journalists outside the convention hall.

Johnson's television campaign in 1964 was extraordinarily effective. His spot ads changed political campaigning. The ads effectively split the Goldwater wing from some of the Rockefeller, Romney and Scranton supporters and the result was a landslide Johnson victory.

The Democrats formed what became known as the "Five O' Clock Club" or "Team D," whose primary purpose was to find something the outspoken Goldwater said and use it against him. Team D also oversaw the creation of some television commercials including the "Daisy Girl" ad. Even though the controversial commercial was aired as a paid advertisement only once, it became a centerpiece of the campaign. Analyzing the ad as news, the television networks provided the Johnson campaign with free replays. Any negative criticism of the president's campaign for "going too far" was offset by the powerful message of the danger of nuclear war. Positive ads developed for Johnson by Team D depicted him as a contemplative, compassionate, concerned and, above all, prudent president. Actor Ronald Reagan appeared in ads on behalf of Goldwater.

Knowing their candidate was ahead, the Democrats were not going to make the mistake Nixon had made by sharing the stage with an acknowledged underdog. The Senate tabled a resolution to suspend Section 315 of the Communication Act of 1934 that would have lifted the requirement to provide equal media time for all the candidates on the ballot. The networks could not undertake the expense of providing broadcast time for all of the candidates, and, therefore, the 1964 campaign held no presidential debates. In addition, the Federal Communications Commission mandated that the equal time provision required a radio or television station that carried a presidential press conference in full to give equal time to other presidential candidates who were on the official ballot. It was to Johnson's benefit, therefore, to remain politically quiescent himself and let surrogates and commercials campaign for him. Goldwater wrote in his memoirs that had President Kennedy lived this aspect of the election might have been different. He and Kennedy had "talked seriously," tentatively agreeing that, if Goldwater was the candidate in 1964, the two would appear "before the same audiences" to discuss their "substantive differences" on the issues.

In 1964, NBC anchors Chet Huntley and David Brinkley were the most watched television news team, and soon other networks would try joint anchors. News reporting was seemingly becoming too big a job for one newscaster. All parts of the campaign, and the conventions in their entirety, were now being covered by all three broadcast networks and nightly newscasts had lengthened from 15 minutes in 1963 to 30 minutes in 1964. The computer-generated results of the November 3 elections were reported by the networks faster than ever before.

THE RESULTS

Lyndon Johnson called his lopsided victory a "mandate for unity." He received 486 electoral votes and 43,129,566 popular votes, or 61.1 percent, the largest percentage of popular votes to this time. Goldwater received 52 electoral votes and 27,178,188 popular votes for 38.5 percent. The Democrats held a 68-seat to 32-seat advantage in the Senate and gained 38 seats in the House for a 295 seat to 140 seat majority. In 1948, Johnson had acquired the nickname "Landslide Lyndon" by winning a Texas Senate race by only 87 votes out of almost a million. He now had a true landslide.

With 45 states, Johnson won big, but fell short of Franklin D. Roosevelt, who won 46 states in 1936. Although he was the first president from the South in almost a century, Johnson failed to hold back a trend that had implications for future elections. With Goldwater victories in Alabama, Georgia, Louisiana, Mississippi and South Carolina, a Republican candidate had once again cracked the Democratic South.

1964

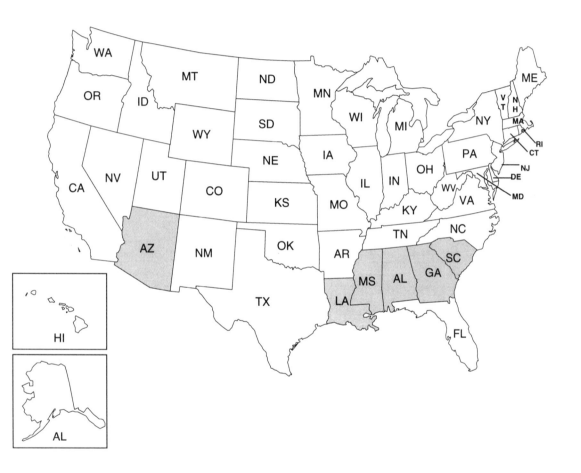

Johnson (Democrat)

Goldwater (Republican)

POSTSCRIPT

In over five years as president, Lyndon Johnson would see much of his Great Society legislation enacted. Because of his knowledge of the legislative process, his proposals, though complex, passed through the legislative branch with more ease than if guided by someone less skilled.

In 1965 alone, he signed the act creating the cabinet-level Department of Housing and Urban Development, established the Department of Transportation and signed the Voting Rights Act of 1965, which provided federal supervision of elections in order to prevent discrimination in voting procedures and registration requirements. President Johnson appointed Thurgood Marshall as the first black justice on the U.S. Supreme Court in 1967. Johnson also presided over increased aid for the public schools and colleges, medical care for the aged and other Great Society legislation. Today, "The Thousand Laws of the Great Society" is a prominent exhibit in the LBJ Library in Austin, Texas.

The fulfillment of Johnson's vision of the Great Society was thwarted by unanticipated problems in Southeast Asia as of 1965. The president soon found that he could not control or escape from the predicament created by the conflict in Vietnam. He tried to keep his domestic agenda on course but found it increasingly difficult to do while fighting a determined enemy in a far-off country. Much of the public responded bitterly to the escalating war because Johnson had said in the campaign that he would not send many more Americans to the conflict. On March 31, 1968, President Johnson announced he would not seek re-election.

"I do not believe that the Great Society is the ordered, changeless, and sterile battalion of the ants.

It is the excitement of becoming—always becoming, trying, probing, falling, resting, and trying again—but always trying and always gaining.

In each generation—with toil and tears—we have had to earn our heritage again.

If we fail now, then we will have forgotten in abundance what we learned in hardship: that democracy rests on faith, that freedom asks more than it gives, and that the judgment of God is harshest on those who are most favored.

If we succeed, it will not be because of what we have, but it will be because of what we are; not because of what we own, but rather because of what we believe."

President Lyndon Baines Johnson
Inaugural Address
January 20, 1965

— 6 —
THE ELECTION OF 1968

*Population of the United States: **200.71 million***
*Number of eligible voters: **120.29 million***
*Percent of those eligible who voted: **60.9***
*Percent of television saturation in U.S. households: **94.6***

SETTING THE STAGE

President Johnson started his term with great ambitions for furthering his Great Society programs, but his domestic agenda was soon muted by the escalation of fighting in Vietnam. News reports of U.S. casualties began to turn public opinion against the war. On January 30, 1968, the North Vietnamese launched a massive offensive in over 30 cities in South Vietnam, including sending Viet Cong "suicide-squads" into Saigon, the capital city. These attacks, labeled the "Tet offensive" by American military leaders, continued unabated until February 24. Ubiquitous and intense television coverage of this bloodshed shocked Americans, whose sense of vincibility and frustration grew. By March 14, the number of American casualties in Vietnam exceeded the total count of the Korean conflict.

Johnson continued to push his two-prong approach to American policy. "I believe we can continue the Great Society while we fight in Vietnam," he claimed. This "guns and butter" strategy strained resources of the federal government, and Johnson soon realized he needed to raise more revenue to bolster the Vietnam war effort. On June 28, he signed a 10 percent income tax surcharge while simultaneously trimming $6 billion in government expenditures.

With the impending presidential election, Johnson soon found that he could not attend to the country's domestic and international crises and still engage in another national election. On March 31, 1968, after the New Hampshire primary and a little over a month after the end of the Tet offensive, President Lyndon Johnson announced that he would not seek re-election.

Another country threatened U.S. security in 1968. On January 23, the North Koreans captured the American intelligence vessel USS *Pueblo*, claiming the ship was within their territorial waters, and did not release the 83-member crew until December 23.

In the spring, the liberalization movement in Czechoslovakia was crushed by the Soviet Union and other Warsaw Pact countries. The same unsettling year, India's Prime Minister Indira Ghandi warned that, unless the gap between the rich and underdeveloped nations was narrowed, "men and women will be impelled to revolt." It was also a year of tumult, protest and violence at home. Outside the White House, protesters relayed antiwar messages to the president by marching and carrying signs with slogans like, "Bombs kill, not demonstrators."

On the civil rights front, a government study called the Kerner Report addressed racism when it warned that the United States was "moving toward two societies, one black, one white, separate and unequal" and called for an end to discrimination. It was submitted by the President's National Advisory Committee on Civil Disorders on February 29. On April 4, 1968, the civil rights movement was dealt a blow when an assassin's bullet took the life of the Reverend Martin Luther King Jr. The civil rights leader had traveled to Memphis, Tennessee, to organize a march of sanitation workers against discriminatory working conditions and was shot on the balcony of his hotel room. That night many took to the streets in protest and civil disturbances arose in major cities around the country. New York Senator Robert Kennedy spoke over the radio trying to calm and reassure an uncomprehending and struggling nation. Two months later, on June 4, in the midst of his presidential campaign, Robert Kennedy was assassinated in Los Angeles, California.

THE CANDIDATES AND THE ISSUES

From the time President Johnson declared he would not seek another term, the election was wide open. Three major candidates emerged; all were well known to the American electorate.

FORMER VICE PRESIDENT RICHARD M. NIXON,
THE REPUBLICAN PARTY CANDIDATE
(Nixon's biography is in chapter four.)

Over the eight years since his defeat by President Kennedy, Richard Nixon had proceeded to rebuild his political support. In 1962, he lost a bitterly fought California governor's contest to Edmund "Pat" Brown. Once again he faced political oblivion. "Gentlemen, this is my last news conference," he said at an emotional press conference. "You'll not have Dick Nixon to kick around anymore." By 1968, Richard Nixon was back.

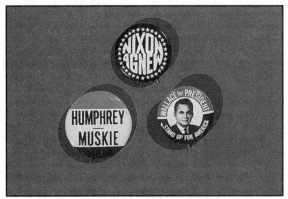

(Campaign materials courtesy private collection of Dr. John Sullivan, University of Virginia/Photo by Paul Kennedy.)

VICE PRESIDENT HUBERT H. HUMPHREY,
THE DEMOCRATIC PARTY CANDIDATE

Humphrey was born on May 27, 1911, in Wallace, South Dakota. He attended the Denver College of Pharmacy and worked as a pharmacist. He graduated from the University of Minnesota in 1939, earned a master's degree from Louisiana State University in 1940 and taught school in Minnesota.

During World War II, Humphrey served as the state director of war production training and re-employment, and chief of the Minnesota

War Service program. He was also assistant director of the War Manpower Commission. From 1943 to 1944 he taught political science at Macalester College. After the war he worked as a radio news commentator. He was elected mayor of Minneapolis in 1945. In 1948 Humphrey ran a successful campaign for the U.S. Senate and won re-election in 1954 and 1960. After losing to John F. Kennedy in the 1960 presidential primaries, Humphrey continued in the Senate until President Johnson chose him as his vice-presidential candidate in 1964.

Hubert H. Humphrey died on January 13, 1978.

FORMER ALABAMA GOVERNOR GEORGE C. WALLACE, THE AMERICAN INDEPENDENT PARTY CANDIDATE

Wallace was born on August 25, 1919, in Clio, Alabama. He graduated from the University of Alabama law school in 1942. He was a flight engineer for the Army Air Forces in World War II. After the war, he practiced law and in 1946 was appointed an assistant attorney general for Alabama. Wallace then served in the Alabama State Legislature from 1947 to 1953. He won election as a state judge and served from 1953 to 1958. Wallace lost his first bid to become Alabama's governor in 1958, but was successful in 1962 and remained in office until 1967, when another term was foreclosed by Alabama law. His wife, Lurleen Wallace, was elected to the next term in the governor's office.

While campaigning for the 1972 Democratic nomination, Wallace was disabled as the result of a gunshot wound. In 1982, Wallace succeeded in a gubernatorial bid and once again served as Alabama's governor. The former governor has continued to speak out on public issues.

◆◆◆

THE ISSUES

Protests against the Vietnam war and demonstrations in favor of civil rights made up the focus of the 1968 campaign. At their national convention in Chicago, Democrats called for a halt to the bombing in Vietnam when it "would not endanger" the Americans still there. As Election Day approached, Hubert Humphrey, who until this juncture had supported President Johnson's approach to the war, changed his position. He began advocating an end to sending American troops to Vietnam and called for their withdrawal as soon as it was feasible to do so. The Republicans were much less divided on the issue.

The war and the draft, inflation and jobs, black activism and the potential of a "white backlash" were all major voter concerns in 1968. Democrats, in particular, were caught in a quandary. They generally supported the administration's social and economic initiatives, but opposed the war in Southeast Asia. This uncertainty about the war resulted in frequent absenteeism at the polls during the primaries and even traditional party supporters were unsure where they stood.

RICHARD M. NIXON, REPUBLICAN

The former vice president, saying he spoke to the issues of the "Great Silent Majority," called for the restoration of order and respect for the law in the United States. He sought solutions for the "crisis of the cities" and advocated a new "war against organized crime" and a crackdown on the drug trade. Nixon said he was dedicated to civil rights. He wanted to reduce taxes, control inflation, balance the budget and share federal revenues with the states. He also favored expanding the role of the vice president.

Nixon advocated a stronger national defense and wanted to end the draft and create a volunteer military after the Vietnam conflict ended. Nixon said he had a plan for achieving an "honorable end to the war."

HUBERT H. HUMPHREY, DEMOCRAT

Campaigning on the initiatives of the Great Society and proposals of his own, the vice president took a strong stand for civil rights and human rights and called for an end to "all the fear that is in our cities."

Humphrey advocated halting the arms race and ending the threat of nuclear war. He said he would continue the negotiations to bring a prompt end to the Vietnam conflict and pledged to obtain "an honorable peace," without a unilateral withdrawal.

GEORGE C. WALLACE, AMERICAN INDEPENDENT

Wallace supported an expanded free-enterprise system and a return to law and order. He wanted to return control of the public schools to the people of every state and end busing for the purpose of school integration. Wallace criticized the civil rights rulings of the Supreme Court and the Great Society legislation of the Johnson administration and said he would take communists "out of every defense plant in the United States."

On international and defense issues, Wallace advocated an expansion of America's "defense capabilities" and a reduction in aid to other countries. He rejected the "no-win strategy" in Vietnam and favored using more military power if the conflict could not be resolved diplomatically.

THE CAMPAIGN

Former Vice President Richard Nixon won the March 12 New Hampshire Republican primary against mainly write-in competition and proceeded to win all the primaries in which he was entered. In California, Nixon strategically opted out of the race, allowing the popular Governor Ronald Reagan to run unchallenged as a favorite son in his home state's primary. It was clear by convention time that Nixon would be the Republican Party candidate for the second time.

The Tet offensive in Vietnam early in the year gave antiwar candidate Eugene McCarthy a midwinter boost in his challenge to his own party's incumbent president. The Minnesota senator was on the ballot in the New Hampshire primary in March, and there made his first inroads against President Johnson. Johnson won a tough write-in campaign, winning over 48 percent of the vote to McCarthy's 42 percent, but McCarthy won more delegates. The fact that an incumbent president was being seriously challenged by a relatively unknown senator drew unprecedented media attention. McCarthy's showing in New Hampshire was enough to alarm Johnson and his advisers that his re-election effort was in political trouble.

On March 31, 1968, 15 days after New York Senator Robert F. Kennedy announced that he too would challenge the president in the primaries, President Johnson said he would not run and told a national television audience that because Americans were fighting in Vietnam and in harm's way, he could not spend his time being a candidate. "I shall not seek and I will not accept the nomination of my party for another term as your President."

In 1964, Robert Kennedy defeated the Republican incumbent, Kenneth Keating, for the U.S. Senate seat from New York. Name recognition alone made him an imposing foe. In joining the 1968 presidential contest, Kennedy found an increasingly crowded field of candidates. Vice President Hubert Humphrey finally added his name on April 27, but he did not compete in the primaries.

Kennedy won primaries in Indiana and Nebraska, but lost to McCarthy in Oregon. He rebounded by winning the South Dakota and the delegate-rich California primaries both on June 4, 1968. Shortly after giving his victory speech in Los Angeles, Robert Kennedy was shot and died two days later.

THE REPUBLICAN NATIONAL CONVENTION, MIAMI BEACH, FLORIDA, AUGUST 5 TO AUGUST 8

Three governors challenged Richard Nixon for the Republican nomination, yet none were able to pose a viable threat. Nelson Rockefeller of New York and Ronald Reagan of California were both considered possible alternatives. Michigan Governor George Romney, early perceived as a potential threat, had planned a significant campaign for the primaries. However, he dropped any plans to run after an ill-received news conference on February 28, in which he suggested he had been "brainwashed" about Vietnam. Thus, any real competition against Nixon had been preempted. In addition, in the eight years since his last presidential candidacy, Richard Nixon had adroitly mended political fences both inside and outside of his party.

The convention nominated former Vice President Richard M. Nixon for president on the first ballot. Maryland Governor Spiro T. Agnew won the vice-presidential nomination.

THE DEMOCRATIC NATIONAL CONVENTION, CHICAGO, ILLINOIS, AUGUST 26 TO AUGUST 29

Perhaps the only period of unity at the Democratic convention was the tribute to the assassinated Robert Kennedy. Just four years earlier at the Atlantic City convention, Robert Kennedy had given an emotional speech in memory of his brother. This time a film honoring the younger Kennedy roused the convention. The impression made on many viewers at home was that in the midst of this, Humphrey appeared to be an afterthought.

The 1968 Democratic convention used more security and had more confrontations with security than any convention since the one in New York in 1924. Protestors outside the Chicago convention hall chanted "The whole world is watching." Students protesting against "Johnson's War" clashed with police, who armed themselves with riot gear and tear gas to fend off the crowd. This chaotic scene was carried on television news programs throughout the country.

Hubert Humphrey, except for surfacing as a write-in candidate, stayed out of the primaries in this race, departing from his campaign tactics of 1960 when he lost the nomination to John Kennedy. Humphrey, Eugene McCarthy and South Dakota Senator George McGovern were all nominated at the convention. Even though Eugene McCarthy had won several primaries, Vice President Humphrey emerged at the convention as the acceptable compromise candidate of the party regulars and was nominated on the first ballot.

Maine Senator Edmund Muskie was chosen as Humphrey's running mate. Inexplicably, the Democrats had chosen both candidates from Northern states even though they needed to attract Southern votes. In the future, the Democrats generally would have to win at least some Southern states in order to win in the Electoral College.

The American Independent Party chose former Alabama Governor George Wallace and retired Air Force General Curtis LeMay of Ohio for their ticket. Talking about the Democratic and Republican nominees, Wallace claimed there was "not a dime's worth of difference between them." LeMay called for a policy toward Vietnam that would "bomb 'em back to the Stone Age." The American Independent Party's nominees would be a factor in the election. They drew over nine million popular votes and won the majority of electoral votes in five states.

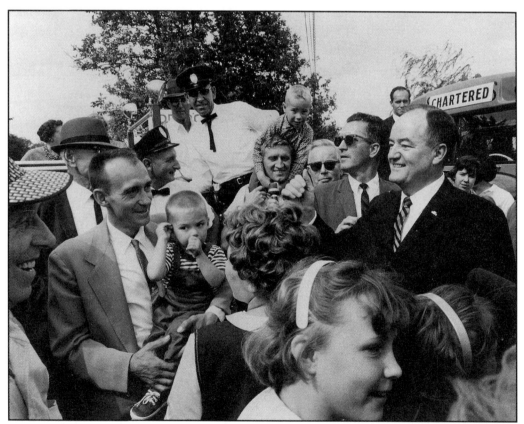

Vice President Hubert H. Humphrey was known as the "Happy Warrior" and campaigned hard before losing his first general election in 20 years.
(Credit:Minnesota Historical Society.)

From the beginning, the election looked as though it was Nixon's to lose, and he ran a guarded campaign until the end when Humphrey tightened the race. Hubert Humphrey, the "Happy Warrior," had not lost a contested general election in 20 years, and he was not about let this election be his political demise without a struggle. Admitting he had an uphill battle, Humphrey worked a hard campaign and by the end he had turned it into a close election.

TELEVISION AND THE CAMPAIGN

In 1968, television continued its march toward becoming an indispensable element of political campaigning, especially in presidential elections. Viewers paid attention to what they saw, and candidates realized that the major networks had the power to affect the political agenda. By 1968, Americans owned 78 million television sets. Advertising revenues for television surpassed $2 billion, about twice the amount brought in by radio advertising.

In 1968, there were still only three major broadcast networks, serving 56.67 million television households. Examples of media influence were increasingly easy to come by, adding to the impact of a medium that was the primary news source for most Americans and the sole news source for some of them. "Walter Cronkite In Vietnam," a CBS News Special, raised questions about American policy; and the fact that the respected Cronkite led the questioning added to the program's impact. At the political conventions, network reporters walking the floor seeking interviews occasionally became part of the story. For example, at the Democratic National Convention in Chicago, Mayor Richard Daley's lieutenants and convention security jostled with several reporters in full view of the television audience. The networks' cameras honed in on the pushing and shoving as the reporters struggled for positions.

Television coverage of violence between police and protestors at the Democratic National Convention did not help the party's image. Connecticut Senator Abraham Ribicoff's denouncement of Mayor

Daley's handling of the demonstrators, on national television, enhanced public perception that both the party and its chosen convention city were in disarray. The power of negative television images would have its effect in the campaign.

Political conventions were now broadcast in color. Good antennas, however, were required for clear reception and for keeping the colors from "bleeding." Richard Nixon used closed-circuit cable television to communicate with delegates, the press and others in various locations at the Republican convention. In 1968, ABC shortened its coverage of the conventions and used edited summaries to report to its audience. Even though CBS and NBC devoted three times more time to the conventions, ABC matched them in the ratings. This suggested to the networks that they could abbreviate their coverage and still satisfy their public obligations.

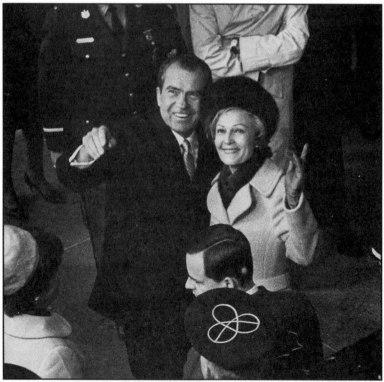

Eight years after losing the general election to John F. Kennedy, Richard M. Nixon won the presidency by defeating Hubert Humphrey by only one percentage point of the popular vote.
(Credit:Consolidated News Pictures/Photo by Gene Forte.)

Nixon and his advisors used television appearances to keep their campaign on track and focused. They carefully selected the television studios and prepped audiences to applaud on cue. These appearances were seeds of the later "electronic town meetings." The Republican choreography paid off against the "unscripted" use of the medium by the Democrats.

The Republicans believed the issues would be favorable to their side and attempted to delineate their positions on the substantive issues of the campaign. They published 167 issue papers, but they realized that more people would look to television for information. At the urging of his aide H. R. Haldeman, Nixon delivered one carefully targeted speech a day. Humphrey, on the other hand, usually made several speeches a day, sending scattered messages. News reporters had a hard time identifying the Humphrey message for their newscasts, but could easily pick up the main points of the single Nixon speech.

Humphrey liked to talk and, like Adlai Stevenson before him, had a tendency to speak too long for television. Humphrey's campaign opener on Labor Day in Detroit's Cadillac Square was scheduled for 20 minutes but went on at least twice that long, ending after some of the crowd and camera crews had gone home. Television as a medium favors visual and personal interaction. Long speeches require a static camera, and reaction shots during these long speeches sometimes catch audience members napping or reading newspapers. The Democrats would soon realize the importance of controlling what images appear on television.

The Democrats and Humphrey wanted televised debates. However, Nixon, careful to avoid any mistakes this time, did not want to debate. Republican Senate leader Everett Dirksen stalled the proposed suspension of the equal time provision, and no presidential debates were held. Humphrey called Nixon's refusal to push for debates characteristic of "Richard the Chickenhearted."

THE RESULTS

Former Vice President Richard Nixon defeated the incumbent Vice President Hubert Humphrey in a hotly contested campaign. The ideological rifts in the Democratic Party, most dramatically seen at the Chicago convention, led to Nixon's capture of normally Democratic middle-class voters. The middle class had been at the center of Franklin D. Roosevelt's political coalition, but was now beginning to lean toward the Republicans in national elections.

Nixon won with only 43.4 percent of the popular vote to Humphrey's 42.7 percent. American Independent George Wallace, running in all 50 states, gained 13.5 percent of the popular vote, a significant showing for a third-party candidate. Wallace's impressive draw indicated that many voters preferred a candidate outside of the two major parties. His hope had been to send the election into the House of Representatives, where he might have brokered a final decision, but Nixon emerged with the necessary majority of electoral votes to win.

The Republicans reduced Democratic strength in the House by seven seats, resulting in 243 Democratic members to 192 Republican members. In the Senate, the Republicans gained five seats, but were still in the minority with a total of 42 seats to 58 Democratic seats.

Nixon defeated Humphrey by less than a percentage point in popular votes and won by 110 votes in the Electoral College. Coming out of a close race, Nixon said in his victory speech that his goal was "to bring the American people together."

1968

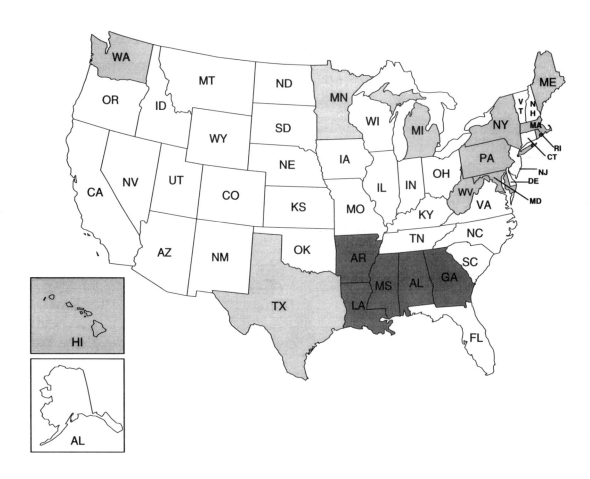

Nixon (Republican)

Humphrey (Democrat)

Wallace (American Independent)

POSTSCRIPT

Nixon's first administration saw relations improve with the Soviet Union and China. The conflict in Vietnam continued; but just before the next election, Nixon again announced he had a plan to end the conflict.

In 1969, the United States and the Soviet Union concurred on strategic arms limitation talks and in May 1972, Nixon, with Leonid Brezhnev, signed the Strategic Arms Limitations Treaty (SALT I). On July 21, 1969, American astronauts Neil Armstrong and Edwin "Buzz" Aldrin became the first men to walk on the moon. Millions watched the historic "first steps" on television. During his first term, Nixon signed federal noise-control regulations, cut taxes $16 billion over three years and imposed wage and price controls.

"For all our people, we will set as our goal the decent order that makes progress possible and our lives secure.

As we reach toward our hopes, our task is to build on what has gone before—not turning away from the old, but turning toward the new.

In this past third of a century, government has passed more laws, spent more money, initiated more programs, than in all our previous history.

In pursuing our goals of full employment, better housing, excellence in education; in rebuilding our cities and improving our rural areas; in protecting our environment and enhancing the quality of life; in all these and more, we will and must press urgently forward.

We shall plan now for the day when our wealth can be transferred from the destruction of war abroad to the urgent needs of our people at home."

President Richard M. Nixon
Inaugural Address
January 20, 1969

= 7 =

THE ELECTION OF 1972

*Population of the United States: **209.9 million***
*Number of eligible voters: **140.78 million***
*Percent of eligible voters who voted: **55.2***
*Percent of television saturation in U.S. households: **95.8***

SETTING THE STAGE

Through 1972, the economy continued to grow, inflation was low, job availability increased and the Dow Jones average rose to 1,000 by November. The downside of the economic news was delivered by President Nixon in the State of the Union Address on January 24: The United States would have its highest peacetime deficit ever, $2.5 billion. Despite this, the home front was considered to be prosperous.

Early in the year, President Nixon traveled to China and Moscow on missions to improve America's relations with these two countries. After the trips, which received substantial television coverage, the president's approval ratings showed a 13-point increase.

Despite this progress in diplomatic affairs, the conflict in Vietnam endured. In fact, it looked as if the conflict might again escalate when the president ordered the mining of Haiphong Harbor and other ports along North Vietnam's coast on May 8, 1972. As Election Day approached, however, Nixon's security advisor, Henry Kissinger, announced that the American commitment in Vietnam would abate. It was hoped that lifting the stigma of Vietnam would place the incumbent in a far better position to win re-election. Even the fervor of antiwar protestors seemed to mellow as the general election approached.

On June 17, 1972, police arrested five men who had broken into the Democratic National Committee headquarters at the Watergate office building in Washington, D.C. At first it appeared that a connection between the break-in and the Republican campaign might be made; but in a news conference on August 29, President Nixon said that an investigation led by White House counsel John Dean had absolved the administration of any involvement.

Assuming he had put the Watergate matter behind him, Nixon moved forward with his campaign, trying to emphasize the accomplishments of his first term. During the year, he signed a bill to share federally collected revenues with the states and local governments, who could then spend their share without significant restrictions. On October 30, he signed a law giving the elderly over $5 billion in added Social Security benefits, which also included a provision extending Medicare to the disabled under age 65. This was on top of a July 1 increase of 20 percent to all Social Security recipients. After much negotiation, the president was able to formalize two strategic arms limitations talks with the Soviet Union. The resulting treaty, SALT I, was favored by the American public and diplomatic leaders not only because it would ease security tensions between the United States and the Soviet Union, but also because many believed the pact would result in a realignment of U.S. government spending priorities from defense programs to domestic areas.

THE CANDIDATES AND THE ISSUES

PRESIDENT RICHARD M. NIXON,
THE REPUBLICAN PARTY CANDIDATE
(Nixon's biography is in chapter four.)

SOUTH DAKOTA SENATOR GEORGE MCGOVERN,
THE DEMOCRATIC PARTY CANDIDATE

McGovern was born in Avon, South Dakota, on July 19, 1922. He graduated from Dakota Wesleyan University in 1945, earned a master's degree in 1949 and a doctorate in history from Northwestern University in 1953. Prior to finishing his education, he served as a pilot in the

Army Air Forces during World War II. After the war he taught at Dakota Wesleyan University.

In 1956, George McGovern was elected to the U.S. House of Representatives and served until he was defeated for re-election in 1960. The following year, he moved back to Washington to head the Food for Peace Program for the Kennedy administration. In 1962, he ran successfully for a seat in the U.S. Senate, and served consecutive terms until 1981. Before retiring, McGovern ran in the presidential primaries of 1984.

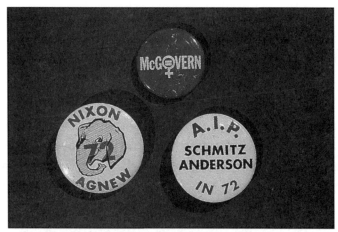

(Campaign materials courtesy private collection of Dr. John Sullivan, University of Virginia/Photo by Paul Kennedy.)

CALIFORNIA REPRESENTATIVE JOHN G. SCHMITZ, THE AMERICAN PARTY CANDIDATE

John Schmitz was born August 12, 1930, in Milwaukee, Wisconsin. He graduated from Marquette University in 1952 and received a master's degree from California State University at Long Beach in 1960.

He taught at Santa Ana College in California and was an aviator in the Marine Corps from 1952 to 1960. Schmitz served in the California State Senate for two terms and in the U.S. House of Representatives from 1970 to 1973. After his run for the presidency, Schmitz wrote *Stranger in the Arena: The Anatomy of An Amoral Decade, 1964-1974*, an account of his political experience.

After retiring from public service, John Schmitz returned to private business.

◆◆◆

THE ISSUES

Democratic candidate George McGovern campaigned for the "immediate and complete withdrawal" of the U.S. military from Vietnam. Nixon said he too wanted to end the war, but only with "honor" and only if the prisoners of war came home along with the troops. In the waning weeks of the campaign, security advisor Kissinger managed to mollify the emotion-laden issues of Vietnam by pledging an end to U.S. participation in the conflict and announcing that the administration had a plan for bringing American soldiers home.

Direct evidence of any Nixon involvement in the Watergate incident was still sketchy and therefore remained a peripheral issue for most voters throughout the campaign.

RICHARD M. NIXON, REPUBLICAN

The president opposed any new taxes and supported full employment as the way to improve the economy and bring more revenue into the federal treasury. He advocated the end of racial discrimination, but opposed hiring quotas and busing efforts to achieve desegregation in schools. Nixon opposed establishing a system for national health insurance and advocated the use of federal moneys to bolster police forces and increase crime prevention efforts. In the campaign, Nixon called his opponent McGovern a "symbol for the liberal culture."

Nixon said he had a plan to end the Vietnam conflict and pledged to recover American POWs still held in Southeast Asia. He supported a strong defense and proposed that future service in the armed forces be strictly voluntary. Emphasizing his strong efforts to ease Cold War tensions, Nixon pledged to continue discussions with China and with the Soviet Union in pursuit of detente.

GEORGE MCGOVERN, DEMOCRAT

McGovern favored a more equitable tax code. He favored a minimum income for both individuals and families and increased public-service employment opportunities. He wanted to put an end to capital punishment and to institute a ban on handguns. He favored school desegregation even if it required court-ordered busing. In the campaign, McGovern alleged deep corruption in the Nixon administration.

McGovern urged the withdrawal of U.S. troops from Vietnam as soon as it was safe to do so. He believed that any future dispatch of U.S. troops for military action abroad should have increased congressional supervision. He favored maintaining America's defensive strength but reducing defense spending.

JOHN G. SCHMITZ, AMERICAN PARTY

Schmitz opposed school busing for desegregation and gun control. He criticized the current welfare system and advocated getting people who could work into a job and off of welfare. Schmitz said that the peace movement included members who were "Stalinists and Trotskyites."

Schmitz campaigned against transferring technology to America's enemies and treating them better than friends at home and abroad. He called for the United States to declare war in Vietnam, to achieve a full victory and to establish a clear intent not to enter future wars with a lesser goal than victory.

THE CAMPAIGN

President Nixon's attorney general, John Mitchell, resigned in February 1972 to head the Committee to Reelect the President (CREEP). He and other campaign leaders had new rules on campaign financing to consider. The new law set by the Federal Election Campaign Act would establish an accounting system for expenditures in presidential campaigns and encourage smaller contributions from more people. Even though the law would not take effect until 1972, reporters were on the alert for any efforts to circumvent its intent in this election.

Nixon, who won easily in the primaries, had only two challengers, Representative Paul N. McCloskey of California and Representative John M. Ashbrook of Ohio. McCloskey, running as an antiwar candidate, won almost 20 percent of the votes in the New Hampshire primary. Overall, Ashbrook won 5 percent of the primary votes and McCloskey won just over 2 percent.

On the other hand, the Democrats, with several strong candidates, had an old-fashioned donnybrook played out in several of the primaries. The media concentrated on the New Hampshire primary, where Senator Edmund S. Muskie of Maine defeated George McGovern, 46 percent to 37 percent, a marginal victory for a candidate from a neighboring state. Muskie's effort may have been hurt by his emotional condemnation of the Manchester Union Leader on February 26, for what he perceived to be an attack on his wife's honor.

Perhaps the most formidable presidential candidate for the Democrats would have been Senator Edward M. "Ted" Kennedy of Massachusetts, youngest brother of the former president. In July 1969, however, the senator's car went off a bridge on Chappaquiddick Island off Cape Cod, Massachusetts. His passenger, Mary Jo Kopechne, was drowned. The ethical questions surrounding the accident and the allegations of special treatment for a member of the Kennedy family rendered a 1972 run for the presidency impossible.

Alabama Governor George Wallace, who had run well in a third-party effort in 1968 and now ran as a Democrat, could have drawn Southern support away from Nixon in the general election. Winning primaries in Florida and Michigan, he further complicated the race for the party regulars, who wanted to unify early behind a candidate. Wallace was making serious inroads into other states when, while campaigning on May 15 in Laurel, Maryland, he was shot and seriously wounded. Wallace was partially paralyzed and discontinued his campaign. At the time, Wallace had 325 primary delegates to McGovern's 405.

Hubert Humphrey could have been a strong opponent in a second run against Nixon, but his campaign faltered when McGovern edged him in the Wisconsin and California primaries. Other entrants at one time or another were Senator Henry Jackson of Washington state, New York Mayor John Lindsay, Representative Shirley Chisholm of New York, former North Carolina Governor Terry Sanford, Representative Wilbur Mills of Arkansas and Los Angeles Mayor Sam Yorty.

THE DEMOCRATIC NATIONAL CONVENTION, MIAMI BEACH, FLORIDA, JULY 10 TO JULY 13

Earlier than anyone had before, McGovern announced on January 18, 1971, that he would be a candidate for president in 1972. McGovern would benefit from a series of campaign rules he had worked on following the 1968 convention. These rules made the Iowa caucuses more important, the primary accumulations a more significant part of the total and reduced the influence of party regulars in the choice of a candidate. The Iowa caucuses, preceding the New Hampshire primary, would soon draw a large share of candidate and, hence, media attention. The importance of early primaries in determining the nominee was magnified by television coverage.

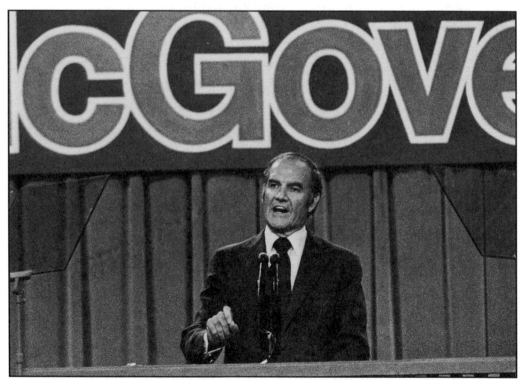

After a protracted fight over the party platform at the Democratic National Convention, Senator George McGovern finally gave his acceptance speech at 2:48 a.m., a time when television viewers were minimal. *(C-SPAN photo.)*

Convention delegates chose McGovern on the first ballot and confirmed Missouri Senator Thomas F. Eagleton as the vice-presidential candidate. After a protracted floor fight and demonstrations over some of the planks in the party platform, McGovern finally gave his acceptance speech at 2:48 a.m. The television viewers at that hour were minimal. Because of the delay, McGovern missed his chance for free, prime time coverage and a large audience. With the increased importance of the primaries and caucuses, the conventions were becoming less decisive and more symbolic. This time the Democratic convention had been symbolic of raw democracy.

The McGovern campaign was unable to recoup any momentum in the weeks to follow. On July 25, McGovern disclosed that Senator Eagleton had been treated for depression. McGovern said that he was "one thousand percent" behind his running mate; but as pressure built to abandon Eagleton, McGovern replaced the nominee with the former director of the Peace Corps, Sargent Shriver of Maryland. As of August 8, it was a McGovern-Shriver ticket.

THE REPUBLICAN NATIONAL CONVENTION, MIAMI BEACH, FLORIDA, AUGUST 21 TO AUGUST 23

Unlike the Democrats, the Republicans were fully united behind their candidates. President Nixon and Vice President Agnew were renominated on the first ballot. The convention was not without controversy, however. On the last day of the gathering, police arrested 1,129 picketers who tried to prevent delegates from entering the convention hall. Many of the protesters had come from nearby Flamingo Park, which had been occupied by the recently formed Vietnam Veterans Against the War, various feminist groups and the participants of Ralph Abernathy's "Poor People's March."

◆◆◆

The euphoria emanating from the unified Republican convention convinced the McGovern campaign that they needed to move fast if they were to defeat Nixon. Television was now the optimal way to increase a candidate's national exposure. To maximize his media opportunities, McGovern traveled extensively in his airplane, the "Dakota Queen II," offering interviews to local and national networks. The advent of "tarmac" campaigning was in its first full swing.

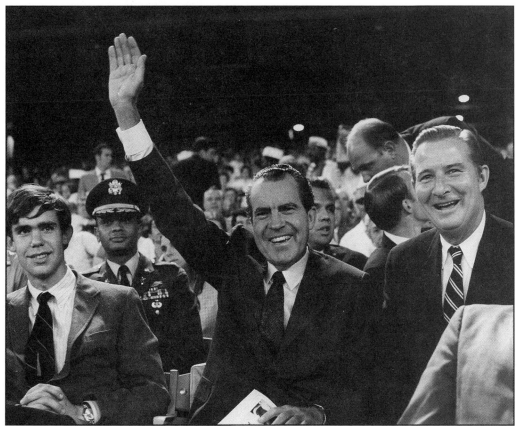

While his Democratic opponent was campaigning, President Nixon stayed close to the White House and performed his presidential duties. *(Credit: Consolidated News Pictures/Photo by Gene Forte.)*

McGovern labeled the Nixon administration "the most corrupt" in the history of the United States. After Labor Day, he tried to pull Democratic Party leaders, whose influence at the convention had been muted, into his camp. But he was not able to open his political tent against the well-run Nixon campaign in time.

Like most powerful incumbents, Nixon had numerous advantages over McGovern. While his Democratic opponent had to declare his candidacy early and campaign longer, Nixon performed his presidential responsibilities, staying close to the White House. Principal stand-ins for the president who canvassed vigorously early in the campaign were Pat Nixon, daughters Tricia and Julie, son-in-law Ed Cox, Vice President Agnew and various cabinet members. In the last three weeks before the election, Nixon was by all indications still well ahead, but he had tired of staying out of the political waters and plunged in. His aides controlled access to the president, carefully selecting and managing his personal appearances. Nixon's main campaign tool was televised speeches.

American Party candidate John Schmitz was on the ballot in 32 states. He criticized the media for not giving him coverage or access equal to the Democratic and Republican party candidates. With over a million votes, he made a respectable third-party showing in the general election.

In retrospect, the 1972 presidential campaign had its share of political espionage and dirty tricks, culminating in the Watergate break-in. On September 15, a federal grand jury indicted the five individuals and two former White House aides who had participated in one way or another in the Watergate incident. *The Washington Post* pursued the story, but the Nixon administration called the reports "a political effort...to discredit this administration and individuals in it." Even the Watergate stories could not derail Nixon's re-election.

TELEVISION AND THE 1972 CAMPAIGN

During a tour in November of 1969, Vice President Spiro Agnew had remonstrated against the power of the news media. He cited distorted coverage in their depiction of public affairs, inaccurate reporting and unfairness toward the administration, and made other charges. "Tonight I want to discuss the importance of the television news medium to the American people," he said. "No nation depends more on the intelligent judgment of the citizens. No medium has a more profound influence over public opinion. Nowhere in our system are there fewer checks on vast power."

Agnew continued, "First, let's define that power. At least 40 million Americans every night, it's estimated, watch the network news. Seven million of them view ABC, the remainder being divided between NBC and CBS. According to the Harris polls and other studies, for millions of Americans the networks are the sole source of national and world news. In Will Rogers' observation, what you knew was what you read in the newspaper. Today for growing millions of Americans, it's what they see and hear on their television sets." His attack on the media struck a powerful chord with some Americans, and not long after the speech, "Spiro, my Hero" bumper stickers appeared.

As late as 1972, there were still only three television networks to divide the audience share. As the Public Broadcasting Service (PBS) was still in its infancy, audiences relied on the commercial broadcast networks to televise the primaries, the conventions, the campaign and the general election. So, the electorate did not have to agree with Agnew's politics to agree with the central thrust of his argument that more choices were desirable.

There were 21 primaries for the television cameras to follow in 1972, and McGovern's good showing in both the Iowa caucuses and the New Hampshire primary gave him what has become known as a "media bump." When a candidate does well or better than expected, the candidacy draws attention resulting in campaign contributions. Since that time, candidates have fought hard in the early contests seeking the "bump."

The power of television also led to reduced influence of political party leaders and the parties themselves. Candidates could now run their campaigns in a more entrepreneurial manner, independent of the party's imprimatur. The early primaries became a litmus test for presidential contenders, and the party leaders discovered that while they still controlled some delegate votes, they were increasingly shut out from wielding influence over primary voters. Their power to select the final nominee was significantly curtailed.

After McGovern's little-viewed, postmidnight speech at the Democratic convention, organizers worked harder at scheduling events especially for television. Campaign aides paid more attention to news deadlines, and pseudo-events were scripted just for the nightly news. Up to 50 million viewers had seen unvarnished democracy displayed at the Democratic convention, and party leaders were going to make sure from then on that the viewers saw the party at its best and heard their candidate's speech in prime time.

Voter turnout for the general election continued to decline to about 55 percent for 1972, enhancing the impact of those who did vote. Ballot counts in the primaries were even lower. As television coverage of the process grew, the early-contest states of Iowa and New Hampshire, although relatively small in population, gained influence on the final outcome.

American Party candidate John Schmitz criticized the media for a "news blackout" of his candidacy. Without equal coverage, it was difficult for a third-party candidate to compete. Although he appeared on programs like CBS's "Face the Nation," Schmitz said that the power of the three networks prevented his message from reaching enough voters.

The powerful attraction of cameras affected post-convention campaigning too. The big media markets were in large cities so McGovern and Shriver would fly to a city's nearest airport, conduct interviews on the tarmac or in the airport lounge, motorcade to television studios for more interviews, shake as many hands as possible upon leaving the studios and then maybe make a quick speech before going to the airport to fly to the next media market.

THE RESULTS

The 26th Amendment to the Constitution, ratified on July 1, 1971, gave the right to vote to citizens 18 years of age and older. Those new voters, ages 18 to 20, voted in lower numbers, replicated the voting patterns of other demographic groups and did not change the outcome in the elections of 1972. The Watergate break-in at the Democratic headquarters also had little impact on the outcome of this election, but it would affect the next election cycle.

The Democrats gained two Senate seats but lost 13 seats in the House of Representatives. The Democratic advantage was now 57 seats to 43 seats in the Senate and 244 seats to 191 seats in the House.

Ten years after telling reporters in California that he had held his "last press conference," Nixon was elected president for the second time. In this election, Nixon won every state but Massachusetts and the District of Columbia. He won the South and a large part of the union vote. Nixon also became the first Republican since exit polling began to win a majority of the Catholic vote.

1972

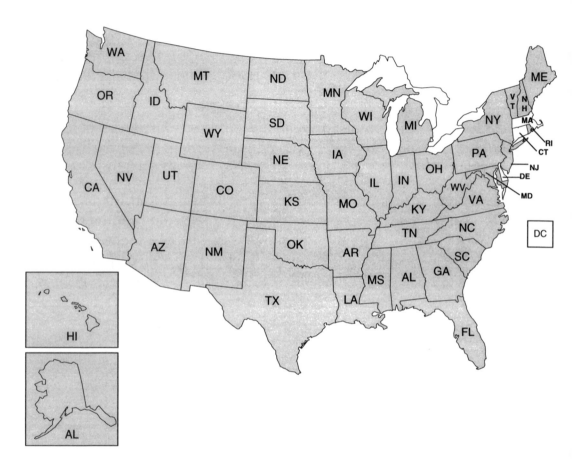

Nixon (Republican)
McGovern (Democrat)

POSTSCRIPT

As he had promised, Nixon ended American participation in Vietnam. The United States signed a cease-fire agreement with the North Vietnamese in 1973, beginning a phased withdrawal of Americans.

As a result of the Nixon administration's role in covering up facts of the break-in of the Democratic National Committee headquarters, the House Judiciary Committee voted on July 30 for three articles of impeachment against President Nixon. With the virtual certainty that the full House would vote for impeachment, resulting in a Senate trial, President Nixon became the first president to end his tenure in office early by resigning, effective at noon on August 9, 1974. Gerald Ford, who replaced Spiro Agnew as vice president, became president of the United States upon Nixon's resignation.

"We have the chance today to do more than ever before in our history to make life better in America—to ensure better education, better health, better housing, better transportation, a cleaner environment—to restore respect for law, to make our communities more livable—and to ensure the God-given right of every American to full and equal opportunity.

Because the range of our needs is so great—because the reach of our opportunities is so great—let us be bold in our determination to meet those needs in new ways.

Just as building a structure of peace abroad has required turning away from old policies that failed, so building a new era of progress at home requires turning away from old policies that have failed.

Abroad, the shift from old policies to new has not been a retreat from our responsibilities, but a better way to peace.

And at home, the shift from old policies to new will not be a retreat from our responsibilities, but a better way to progress.

Abroad and at home, the key to those new responsibilities lies in the placing and the division of responsibility. We have lived too long with the consequences of attempting to gather all power and responsibility in Washington."

President Richard M. Nixon
Second Inaugural Address
January 20, 1973

= 8 =
THE ELECTION OF 1976

Population of the United States: **218.04 million**
Number of eligible voters: **152.31 million**
Percent of eligible voters who voted: **53.5**
Percent of television saturation in U.S. households: **97**

SETTING THE STAGE

By the end of President Gerald Ford's term, the American withdrawal from Vietnam was complete and no U.S. troops were in combat anywhere in the world. After the crises of the late 1960s and early 1970s, the nation longed for stability, and the conciliatory style of the new president helped "heal" the American spirit. During most of 1973 and early 1974, people watched the Watergate investigation unfold on television. The volatility of Vietnam, the Watergate hearings and the resignations of the nation's two top officials had made for turbulent times. At this point, the nation was ready for a respite.

Vice President Spiro T. Agnew resigned his office on October 10, 1973, after pleading no contest to charges of tax evasion during his service as governor of Maryland. Two days after Agnew's resignation, President Nixon appointed House Minority Leader Gerald R. Ford of Michigan to be vice president, the first appointment made under provisions of the 25th Amendment, ratified in 1967. Ford had served in Congress since 1949, and as minority leader since 1965. Both houses of Congress confirmed the appointment, voting 479 to 38.

As a result of the vote on articles of impeachment, President Nixon announced his resignation, effective at noon August 9, 1974. As ex-President Nixon left for California, Gerald Ford took the oath of office and became the first person ever to assume the presidency without having been directly elected by the people. President Ford, also acting under the 25th Amendment, appointed former New York Governor Nelson R. Rockefeller as his vice president.

President Ford was more than a caretaker president. In his first 21 months in office, he vetoed 48 bills. He issued a presidential amnesty for draft evaders and military deserters during the Vietnam war. In 1974, he established diplomatic relations with East Germany. On September 8, 1974, he gave former President Nixon an unconditional pardon for any federal crimes he may have committed in office. It was

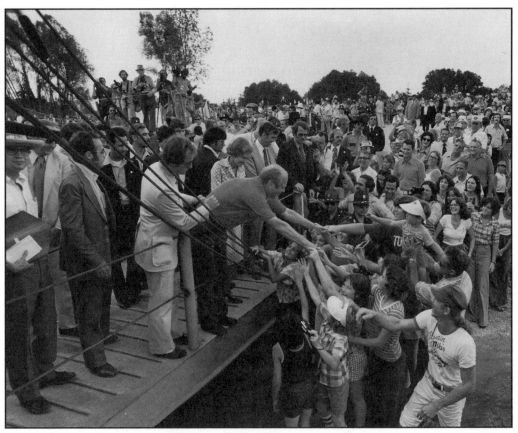

Gerald Ford campaigned hard in 1976. He was the only man to be appointed, not elected, to both the vice presidency and the presidency.
(Courtesy Gerald R. Ford Library.)

his most controversial act, according to the reactions of a still-recovering public and a wary press. In April 1975, Ford presided over the removal of the last embassy personnel from South Vietnam before it surrendered to the communists and said on April 30 that Americans could now "look ahead to the many goals we share and...the great tasks that remain to be accomplished."

In the election year of 1976, President Ford signed the Railroad Revitalization and Reform Act, which authorized $6.4 billion for railroads and appropriated $2.14 billion in additional funds to complete the Northeast Corridor from Washington through New York and up to Boston. In the two years and 164 days of his administration, Gerald Ford also presided over a recession, high inflation and oil shortages. The inflation rate hovered between 5 percent and 6 percent and unemployment was close to 8 percent at various times.

Internationally, President Ford responded quickly to the Cambodian seizure of American merchant ship *Mayaguez* and secured its release on May 14, 1974. Though America was not at war, sporadic unrest throughout the world continued to affect the United States. On June 16, 1976, the worst racial violence in South Africa's history began in Soweto and spread to other townships. Almost 200 people were killed and over 1,000 people injured. Also in 1976, the Mexican government devalued the peso, the result of the previous year's economic instability—a $3.7 billion trade deficit and an inflation rate fluctuating between 40 percent and 50 percent. Mexico's economic problems had an impact on U.S. and other international markets.

THE CANDIDATES AND THE ISSUES

If political pundits had been asked in 1972 or 1973 who would be the Democratic and Republican nominees in 1976, few would have chosen Gerald Ford or foreseen Jimmy Carter's ascension to national politics. Yet, as is often the case in American politics, surprise often defines the predictions game.

FORMER GEORGIA GOVERNOR JAMES EARL "JIMMY" CARTER JR., THE DEMOCRATIC PARTY CANDIDATE

Carter was born October 1, 1924, in Plains, Georgia, the first U.S. president to be born in a hospital. When he was four, his family moved to a farm in nearby Archery, where he spent the rest of his childhood. He married Eleanor Rosalyn Smith on July 7, 1946. The couple had one daughter, Amy Lynn, and three sons, John "Jack," James "Chip" and Donnell Jeffrey.

Jimmy Carter graduated from the U.S. Naval Academy in 1946 and became the first graduate to later become president of the United States. In his shortened naval service, he reached the rank of lieutenant senior grade. Carter's naval career was cut short by the death of his father in 1953. Carter then left the Navy and returned to Plains to manage his family's peanut farm and business interests.

Before running for the Georgia legislature, Carter was chairman of the Sumter County Board of Education and active in other local civic affairs. He was elected to the State Senate in 1962 and served until 1967. After a failed attempt in 1966, Carter won the governorship in 1970. Georgia state law prevented him from running for a second term in 1974.

After serving as president, Carter moved back to Plains, Georgia, and wrote several books.

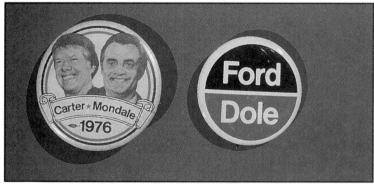

(Campaign materials courtesy private collection of Dr. John Sullivan, University of Virginia/Photo by Paul Kennedy.)

PRESIDENT GERALD R. FORD JR.,
THE REPUBLICAN PARTY CANDIDATE

Ford was born on July 14, 1913, at his family's home in Omaha, Nebraska. He married Elizabeth "Betty" Bloomer Warren on October 15, 1948. The couple had one daughter, Susan Elizabeth, and three sons, Michael Gerald, John "Jack" and Steven Meigs.

Ford graduated from the University of Michigan in 1935 and the Yale law school in 1941. He practiced law until he joined the Navy. Serving in the Pacific during World War II, he advanced to the rank of lieutenant commander.

Ford was elected to the U.S. House of Representatives in 1948 and served in that body continuously until 1973. The Republicans selected him as their minority leader in 1965. In 1973 President Nixon appointed him vice president after the resignation of Spiro Agnew. Ford then assumed the presidency upon Nixon's resignation. He was the only person to serve as vice president and president without being elected to either office.

After the 1976 election, Ford returned to private life, retiring to Rancho Mirage, California.

◆◆◆

THE ISSUES

Jimmy Carter campaigned as a "populist" against the entrenched powers in Washington. He used the fact that he had never held elected office in the U.S. capital as proof that he was not "one of them," an appeal to a citizenry that had become distrustful of Washington insiders. He said that if elected he would take steps to curb the high rate of inflation, to improve employment opportunities and to address the other economic challenges facing American families. He wanted to make government more efficient, and he condemned the Republican Party for its scandals and criticized the incumbent administration for its pardon of Nixon and its "lack of leadership."

President Ford, on the other hand, boasted that recent Republican administrations had ended U.S. involvement in Vietnam and that Republicans had made the world a safer place to live in 1976. In a September 17 speech at his alma mater, the University of Michigan, he said, "Today America enjoys the most precious gift to all: we are at peace. No Americans are in combat anywhere on earth, and none are being drafted—and I will keep it that way." In addition to campaigning on a peace plank, Ford claimed credit for America's general prosperity and pledged to make it even better. "Today 88 million Americans are gainfully employed—more than ever before in our history. But that's not good enough."

Despite these pledges, Ford was unable to prevent a downturn in the economy. The U.S. unemployment rate had risen to 8 percent, and Ford's economic recovery program, Whip Inflation Now (WIN), had been unsuccessful in lowering either the unemployment or the inflation rates. The anomalous presence of high inflation coinciding with high unemployment introduced a new word into the economic vocabulary: "stagflation."

JIMMY CARTER, DEMOCRAT

Carter favored an overhaul of the income tax system and a balanced federal budget. He wanted to make the government more competent and efficient, calling for the reorganization of the executive branch. Carter guaranteed an end to discrimination, advocated universal voter registration and, if necessary to desegregate the schools, he would support the use of busing. Carter supported gun control, spoke out against the proposed "Right to Life" amendment and wanted a comprehensive national health system.

Jimmy Carter took a strong stand for worldwide human rights and favored agreements among nations extending such protections to their citizens. He wanted to reduce the defense budget while still standing firm against the Soviet Union. He pushed for a mutually acceptable Panama Canal treaty that took into consideration the concerns of Latin American countries.

GERALD R. FORD, REPUBLICAN

The incumbent president wanted to reduce the growth and cost of government and return governmental control to the states and localities. He planned to submit a balanced budget by 1978.

Ford wanted to make government more efficient, to cut taxes and raise personal exemptions and to provide incentives for economic investment. He opposed national health insurance and gun control and proposed amending the Constitution to restrict court-ordered busing and ban abortion.

Ford called for increased defense spending and wanted to keep the Panama Canal under U.S. control.

THE CAMPAIGN

At the beginning of the campaign, it looked as if the Democratic nominee might be Senator Henry "Scoop" Jackson of Washington state or even a long shot like Alabama Governor George Wallace, who had done well as a third-party candidate in 1968. Knowing his disadvantage as a newcomer, Jimmy Carter, the former governor and farmer from Georgia, started early and campaigned hard. He announced his candidacy almost two full years before the election, in December 1974, and made frequent trips to Iowa and New Hampshire in preparation for the caucuses and primaries.

Carter finished second in the Iowa caucuses, winning 29.1 percent of the vote behind the 38.5 percent for the category marked "uncommitted." But "uncommitted" could not be interviewed and Carter could, thus providing the governor the limelight. Carter won New Hampshire with 28 percent of the vote, edging Arizona Representative Morris Udall, who had 22 percent. Henry Jackson took Massachusetts, but Carter won 17 of the 26 remaining primaries. He was well on his way to the nomination. After his win in New Hampshire, both Time and Newsweek put Carter on their covers, an exposure that helped propel him to victory in the other states. Carter had risen quickly from political obscurity to victory in over half of the primaries he entered. His fast start brought him valuable media attention. California Governor Edmund G. "Jerry" Brown Jr. entered the May 18 Maryland primary, winning there, in Nevada and in California. But at this stage, it was too late to stop Carter.

Although the Republicans had an incumbent president, they still had a contest. Ronald Reagan, the former governor of California, mounted a serious challenge. Ford won the New Hampshire primary by little over a percentage point. Reagan won the much more populous delegation of California, his home state. By the time the Republicans met in their national convention Ford had 53.3 percent of the votes from the primaries and Reagan had 45.9 percent. Ford won 15 primaries to Reagan's 10.

THE DEMOCRATIC NATIONAL CONVENTION, NEW YORK, NEW YORK, JULY 12 TO JULY 15

Jimmy Carter had won a sufficient number of delegates during the primaries to be assured of a first ballot victory. The convention then confirmed Senator Walter Mondale of Minnesota as Carter's running mate. Keynote speeches were given by Senator John Glenn of Ohio, a former astronaut, and Representative Barbara Jordan of Texas, who was the first black woman to deliver a convention floor address. The national party then unified behind the proclaimed "outsider," whose unassuming self-introduction in his acceptance speech won over the crowd. "My name is Jimmy Carter and I am running for president."

THE REPUBLICAN NATIONAL CONVENTION, KANSAS CITY, MISSOURI, AUGUST 16 TO AUGUST 19

The Republicans gathered in the country's midsection for their meeting. Reagan continued to challenge Ford at the convention. Both candidates arrived three days early to battle for delegate support. Ford prevailed, winning on the first ballot by 117 votes out of a total of 2,257 delegate ballots cast. Ford then chose Senator Robert Dole of Kansas to complete the ticket. In his acceptance speech, Ford challenged Carter to debate saying, "The American people have the right to know where both of us stand."

Throughout the campaign, Carter reminded people that Ford had been part of the Nixon administration. Carter vowed, "I'll never tell a lie; I'll never make a misleading statement." Running against both Ford and Nixon and identifying their Washington centricity as the crux of problems in the federal government, Carter turned his lack of Washington experience into an asset.

To reinforce his base in small-town America and his middle-class values, Carter and his advisers decided to use his hometown, Plains, Georgia, as a "television studio." Carter, the campaigner, was on the go from dawn to dusk, leaving the red clay country of Georgia early on his campaign plane, "Peanut One." Carter met people door-to-door and gradually built up his "Peanut Brigade" of supporters.

Carter steadily moved ahead of Ford in the polls until the November issue of Playboy magazine hit the newsstands early. It featured a broad interview with Carter in which he said he had experienced lust in his heart. The political issues discussed were lost amid the media attention and public discussion of that statement. According to Patrick Caddell, Carter's chief pollster, Carter dropped 10 points in the polls after the magazine came out. Ford soon drew into a virtual tie.

As a Washington outsider, Carter benefited from changes to the Federal Elections Campaign Act of 1971 (FECA), particularly from the federal matching funds for eligible candidates, made available by a 1974 FECA amendment. New election finance laws also applied limits on personal and corporate campaign contributions, opening the door for Political Action Committees (PACs) to offer funds.

For the first time since Nixon and Kennedy in 1960, the presidential candidates met in debate. Ford knew he was behind in the polls and took the unusual step for an incumbent of pressing for the meetings with his lesser-known opponent. The candidates debated three times on national television. The second encounter yielded a comment that the Carter camp made into political hay: Ford said there was "no Soviet domination of Eastern Europe." Carter countered, "I'd like to see Mr. Ford convince the Polish-Americans that they [Poland] are not under Russian domination." Standing on the same dais as the president, Carter's strong response helped him gain the stature he needed. The American people were beginning to believe that a one-time governor from Georgia could do the job and were warming to the idea of a maverick as president.

During his campaign, beginning in December 1974, Carter made 1,495 speeches, traveled over 500,000 miles and visited over 1,000 cities. Ford, who traveled less, used a campaign train in Illinois called the "Honest Abe." Both Betty Ford and Rosalyn Carter were active and popular campaigners.

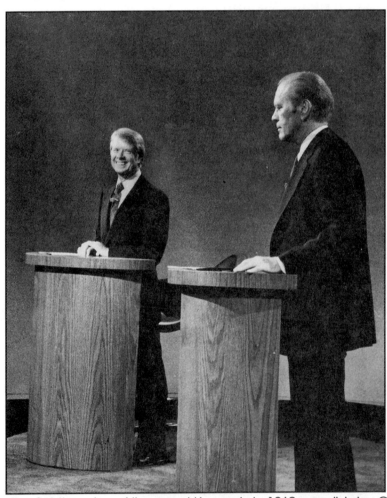

In 1976, for the first time since Nixon and Kennedy in 1960, candidates Gerald Ford and Jimmy Carter met for three televised presidential debates.
(Courtesy The League of Women Voters Archives.)

Jimmy Carter campaigned on issues like reforming the income tax system, reorganizing the federal government, curbing inflation and creating more good jobs. He called for a "New Generation of Leadership" and asked for a chance to demonstrate it.

Ford initially tried a modified "rose garden" strategy, similar to the "front porch" campaigns of 1896 and 1920 in which William McKinley and Warren G. Harding, respectively, campaigned in front of their homes, while the Republican Party sent surrogates around the country to gain votes. Ford's campaign team concluded that he needed to win five pivotal states and that is where he targeted his energies. Once President Ford decided to emerge from the White House and challenge Carter, he concentrated on California, Illinois, Michigan, New Jersey, New York, Ohio, Pennsylvania and Texas. He won four of these eight states in the general election.

◆◆◆

Television and the 1976 Campaign

In 1976, televised presidential debates became a part of the campaign fabric. ABC, CBS and NBC all carried the debates to large audiences. In September of 1975, the FCC held that broadcast political debates qualified as on-the-spot news coverage and were exempt from equal time provisions if sponsored by an independent organization and if covered contemporaneously. Therefore, in 1976, for the first time since 1960 and only the second time in history, the presidential candidates debated on nationwide television. The format of the 1976 debates, sponsored by the League of Women Voters, included a moderator and three panelists to question the candidates. In addition, candidates for vice president debated on television for the first time ever when Walter Mondale and Robert Dole met on October 10.

In the first Ford-Carter debate on September 23, there was a 27-minute audio breakdown. The candidates at this point were so schooled in television technique that they knew to keep their eyes trained on the camera lest it catch them looking distracted. Ford's so-called gaffe in the second debate on October 6 was actually more complicated than reported. Even Eastern Europeans would admit to the nuances contained in his statement regarding the Soviet Union's control over their affairs, but these complexities were hard to explain in a two-minute response and the news media picked up on the brief statement. The last debate, on October 22, was mostly a restatement of previous positions.

By 1976, the candidates had identified a "television uniform"— navy-blue suit, red tie and an off-white shirt that would not glare under the television lights. They now routinely used television makeup for appearances and were professionally coached to be casual, conversational and cool for the cameras.

In 1976, the Democrats were determined to put on a better convention show than their opponents. The parties by now had recognized the advantages of operating their own lighting in the rented convention halls. When Carter entered Madison Square Garden, the spotlight stayed on him and the television cameras had to go where the lights were. The party spent $200,000 to improve lighting at the convention. Campaign workers also needed to restrain the ubiquitous hand-held camera that could now roam the floor. They knew that until low-light technology became more sophisticated, controlling the lighting was the best way to control the images broadcast from the convention.

Both Carter and Ford understood the power of symbols. Carter used Plains, Georgia, as a television stage and Franklin Roosevelt's home in Warm Springs, Georgia, as the setting to open his campaign. The photo-opportunity site for Ford, the White House Rose Garden, was called by a newscaster, "the greatest set television ever had."

Television commercials for Ford sought discreetly to mute the Watergate issue, downplay his position as an appointed president and emphasize his good character: "He's making us proud again."and "Without seeking the presidency, Gerald Ford has been preparing for it all his life." Republican ads portrayed Carter as "wishy-washy."

Carter's flashy, but friendly, smile, was an advantage on television. His appearance and low-tech commercials reinforced his image as "anti-slick," contrasting him to the unctuous Washington-types he was avowedly running against. The Carter commercials focused on his return to the land where his father had lived and died and showed how, as manager of the family's business, he sifted peanuts alongside other farm workers. As Election Day approached, television commercials from both sides hit the airwaves as often as their campaign resources allowed.

THE RESULTS

Jimmy Carter, former governor of Georgia, won four large industrial states, his base in the South and gained enough of the rest of the nation to be elected the 39th President of the United States on November 2, 1976.

Voters gave Carter only 57 more electoral votes than they gave Ford; a shift in just one or two big industrial states would have thrown the election the other way. As anticipated, Kansas Senator Dole helped President Ford carry the farm states and the West. But Ford's sweep of the Western states was not enough. Carter became the first president elected from the "deep" South since Zachary Taylor in 1848. The Georgian's national victory heralded a renewed influence for the increasingly populous South. Democratic Party loyalty had been a Southern tradition, but in recent elections it had not been taken for granted. Carter's roots in Georgia proved decisive in this election.

In winning, Carter reunited most of the old Democratic coalition: labor, large cities, northern Catholics, some key farm states and most of the South and blacks. Over 90 percent of black voters had supported Carter. He also added a good portion of Southern Baptists, who thought of him as one of their own.

Carter might have earned a bigger victory had he won California's large number of electoral votes. California Governor Jerry Brown, a fellow Democrat who had challenged Carter in the primaries, did not campaign for him in the state. President Ford won California's 45 electoral votes by less than 2 percentage points. Carter faulted himself

1976

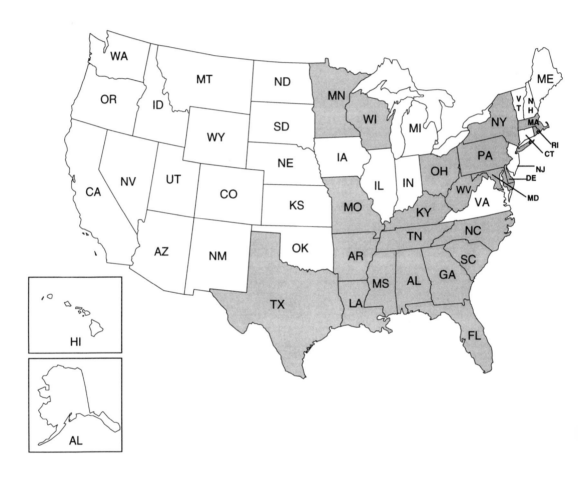

Carter (Democrat)

Ford (Republican)

for failing to win a bigger victory. "The only reason it was close was that I as a candidate was not good enough as a campaigner. But I'll make up for that as president."

The Democrats again won the Congress. They held the House of Representatives, 292 seats to 143 seats. In the Senate there were 62 Democrats and 38 Republicans. If the Senate's Democrats held together, they would be filibuster-proof.

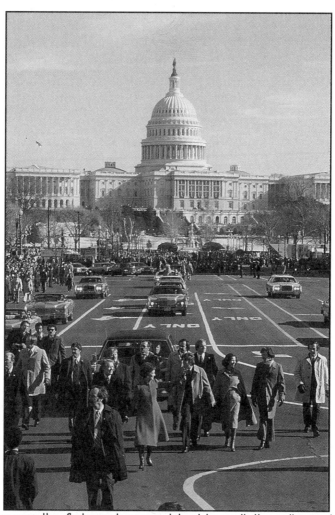

Jimmy Carter was the first modern president to walk the mile and a half down Pennsylvania Avenue from the Capitol to the White House after the inaugural ceremony. *(Credit: Consolidated News Pictures/Photo by Ron Sachs.)*

POSTSCRIPT

Jimmy Carter was the first modern president to walk the mile and a half down Pennsylvania Avenue from the Capitol to the White House after his inauguration.

President Carter wanted to make a government "as good...and honest...as the American people." In 1977, he presided over the creation of the Department of Energy and signed the Panama Canal Zone treaties for the gradual transfer of the area to Panama. In 1978, he mediated private talks between Egyptian President Anwar Sadat and Israeli Prime Minister Menachem Begin at Camp David, Maryland. The two nations, for the first time, agreed to peace and signed the "Camp David Accords." Carter also opened full diplomatic relations with China in 1979. In 1978, the president signed a bill deregulating the commercial airline industry and approved deregulation of natural gas prices. In 1980 he approved deregulation of the trucking industry. Carter signed a bill on October 17, 1979, that elevated the Department of Education to cabinet level.

"Let our recent mistakes bring a resurgent commitment to the basic principles of our Nation, for we know that if we despise our own government we have no future. We recall in special times when we have stood briefly, but magnificently, united. In those times no prize was beyond our grasp.

But we cannot dwell on remembered glory. We cannot afford to drift. We reject the prospect of failure or mediocrity or an inferior quality of life for any person. Our Government must at the same time be both competent and compassionate.

We have already found a high degree of personal liberty, and we are now struggling to enhance equality of opportunity. Our commitment to human rights must be absolute, our laws fair, our natural beauty preserved; the powerful must not persecute the weak, and human dignity must be enhanced."

President James E. Carter
Inaugural Address
January 20, 1977

= 9 =

THE ELECTION OF 1980

Population of the United States: **227.73 million**
Number of eligible voters: **164.6 million**
Percent of those eligible who voted: **52.6**
Percent of television saturation in U.S. households: **98**

SETTING THE STAGE

As a result of the 1980 Census, the South and the West gained 17 seats in the House of Representatives, taking them from the Northeast and the Midwest. The reapportionment moved seats from traditionally more liberal industrial states to more conservative areas of the nation.

President Carter already had his hands full in 1980 with high unemployment rates (7.1 percent), high inflation (13.5 percent) and high interest rates. The Federal Reserve had increased the discount rate to 13 percent, and by December 19 it would be 21.5 percent. On March 31, 1980, President Carter signed a bill deregulating the banking industry hoping that it would spur positive economic activity.

The United States also faced mounting international problems, particularly as tensions with the Soviet Union escalated in the aftermath of the Afghanistan invasion in December 1979. Along with 63 other nations, the United States decided to boycott the 1980 Summer Olympics scheduled for July in Moscow. Judging from the dismay at home and abroad, it was a no-win decision for Carter.

Communist countries that had long been under the influence of the Soviet Union finally began to take steps to move away from even peripheral hegemony. In August, Lech Walesa, a 37-year-old electrician, led Poland's Solidarity Movement in organizing the first labor union in a country under the Soviet sphere. War between Iran and Iraq started in 1980 and would last until 1989, resulting in instability on the Soviet Union's southwest border.

On November 4, 1979, more than 500 Iranian students seized 90 hostages at the U.S. Embassy in Teheran and set off a prolonged diplomatic stalemate for Carter as he entered the election year. The United States completely severed relations with the Iranian government on April 7, 1980. Frustrated by lack of resolution in the crisis, Carter ordered a military rescue of the hostages in a raid later in April. This raid was a failure that cost eight American lives while the hostages remained in Iran. Secretary of State Cyrus Vance, who had opposed the ill-fated mission, resigned in protest.

In this election year, crime, including white-collar crime, was becoming an even more important issue for the American public. The violent killings of several well-known people served to highlight the crime issue in the news media. Ex-congressman Allard Lowenstein was shot and killed in his New York office by a former associate. Musician John Lennon was shot and killed outside his New York apartment. Jean Harris, the head of the Madeira school in Virginia, killed Dr. Herman Tarnower, renowned author of the Scarsdale diet book, during a lover's quarrel. Michael Halberstam, prominent physician and author, was killed by a burglar during a break-in at his home in Washington, D.C.

◆◆◆

THE CANDIDATES AND THE ISSUES

FORMER CALIFORNIA GOVERNOR RONALD REAGAN, THE REPUBLICAN PARTY CANDIDATE

Reagan was born February 6, 1911, in Tampico, Illinois. He married Sara Jane Fulks (the actress Jane Wyman) on January 6, 1940. The couple had one daughter, Maureen, and an adopted son, Michael. They divorced in 1948. On March 4, 1958, Reagan married Anne Francis

"Nancy" Davis, also an actress. They had a daughter, Patti Davis, and a son, Ronald Prescott.

Reagan graduated from Eureka College in Illinois in 1932 and worked as a sportscaster for WHO radio station in Des Moines, Iowa, from 1932 to 1937. Reagan started acting in the film "Love Is in the Air." He was a captain in the Army Air Forces in World War II and made training films. After the war, Reagan continued his acting career, becoming politically active in the Screen Actors Guild and serving as its head from 1947 to 1952 and again in 1959. He was also a national advertising spokesman for the General Electric Company from 1952 to 1962.

In 1962 Reagan switched from the Democratic Party to the Republican Party. He ran successfully for governor of California in 1966, won re-election in 1970 and held the office until 1975. In 1969, he chaired the Republican Governors' Association. He challenged Gerald Ford for the presidential nomination in the 1976 Republican primaries.

After serving two terms as president, from 1980 to 1988, Reagan retired to California and continued to give speeches and advice on public policy matters.

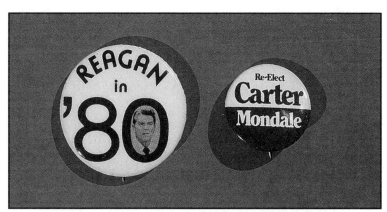

(Campaign materials courtesy private collection of Dr. John Sullivan, University of Virginia/Photo by Paul Kennedy.)

PRESIDENT JAMES EARL CARTER JR.,
THE DEMOCRATIC PARTY CANDIDATE
(President Carter's biography is in chapter eight.)

ILLINOIS REPRESENTATIVE JOHN B. ANDERSON,
INDEPENDENT CANDIDATE

Anderson was born on February 5, 1922. He was an Illinois state attorney from 1959 to 1960. In 1960, he ran successfully for the U.S. House of Representatives as a Republican and served continuously from 1961 to 1980.

After the election, Anderson returned to private life where he continued to speak out on public issues.

THE ISSUES

By 1980, many Americans believed that government was not working well and a large number blamed the incumbent President Jimmy Carter. Ironically, Carter was now the Washington insider and his challenger Ronald Reagan entered the race campaigning against the shortcomings of the federal government, just as Carter had four years earlier.

Both Anderson and Reagan reproached Carter for the state of the economy. The president had promised the American people he would not lie to them and would not claim that things were better than they actually were.

While international affairs had been tangential to the 1976 campaign, they came to the fore in 1980. Carter's response to the hostage crisis demonstrated, for some, his weakness as a president. It also cast doubts that he could fulfill his promise from the 1980 State of the Union speech to keep oil flowing through the Persian Gulf. The Iranian situation and the energy crisis of the 1970s made the American people realize that turmoil abroad could jeopardize oil supplies at home.

RONALD REAGAN, REPUBLICAN

Reagan campaigned for a return to the "American spirit of volunteer service." He called for teaching children values at school and at home. He pledged that the federal government should work for the people, not the other way around. Looking to eliminate "needless regulation" and find measures to spur "real" economic growth, he proposed a citizen task force "to rigorously examine every department and agency." Reagan pledged to reduce income taxes 30 percent over three years, while at the same time lowering the deficit and balancing the budget. He advocated a constitutional amendment to ban abortion and opposed a system of national health insurance.

On international issues, Reagan advocated higher defense spending and the development of a missile defense shield (the Strategic Defense Initiative). He supported the Afghan rebels opposing the Soviet occupation and pressed for release of the hostages in Iran. He opposed ratification of SALT II, which included a ban on all new intercontinental ballistic missiles (ICBMs), unless significant alterations were made.

Jimmy Carter, Democrat

Carter continued his defense of human rights. He called for equal rights for all and appropriate laws to help eradicate discrimination from American society. The president wanted to create good jobs through both public and private efforts and to provide aid to higher education and make quality education available to everyone. He favored a national health insurance. Carter supported ratification of the Equal Rights Amendment and opposed a constitutional amendment banning abortion.

President Carter wanted to guarantee peace through American "military and moral strength." He supported strengthening American defenses and continued negotiations on SALT II with the Soviet Union.

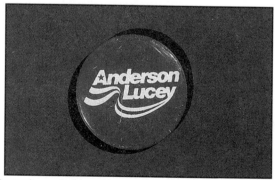

(Campaign materials courtesy private collection of Dr. John Sullivan, University of Virginia/Photo by Paul Kennedy.)

John Anderson, Independent

Anderson identified a "domestic economic decline" and campaigned for a common-sense economic policy to replace "the charade" of the present government's efforts to restrain wage and price increases. He proposed specific tax reductions that he hoped would rebuild the economy, including a lower Social Security tax. He opposed a constitutional amendment banning abortion.

The congressman advocated an increase in gasoline taxes to reduce consumption and lessen American reliance on imported oil. He favored a strong national defense and the ratification of SALT II.

The Campaign

At the start of the primary season, the Republicans knew they had a good shot against a seemingly vulnerable incumbent president and they had many contenders to choose from. Initially, the candidates included John Connally, a Democrat and formerly a governor of Texas; former CIA director George Bush; Senator Robert Dole of Kansas; Senator Howard H. Baker of Tennessee; Representative Philip Crane of Illinois, Representative John B. Anderson of Illinois and former California Governor Ronald Reagan, who, prior to becoming a Republican, had campaigned for Harry Truman.

With James A. Baker III managing his campaign, George Bush started out with a well-coordinated effort and won the Iowa caucuses against Reagan. Reagan, who had declined to campaign in Iowa or to debate Bush, did not show the same reticence in New Hampshire. He even bought time in a debate administered by the Nashua Telegraph *that was well covered by the media. During an ensuing dispute over the rules for who could participate, Reagan was cut off by moderator Jon Breen. Reagan responded sharply, "I'm paying for this microphone, Mr. Green [sic]." Despite the error, the quick, cogent response and the applause of the audience played well on the nightly news. The debate went on with the focus mainly on the give and take between Bush and Reagan. Reagan took the offensive early and kept the pressure on and Bush was left to defend himself.*

There was intense media attention on the New Hampshire primary, augmenting its importance. Reagan won there against Bush, getting an early "media bump," and was on his way to the nomination. Reagan ended the primary season with 28 wins to Bush's five. Bush withdrew on May 26 and endorsed the Reagan candidacy.

Despite having an incumbent president in the race, the Democrats also had contested primaries. Three days after the Iranians took American hostages in Teheran, Senator Edward M. Kennedy of Massachusetts announced that he would challenge Carter for the nomination. Governor Jerry Brown of California, who had tried to stop Carter in 1976, also wanted the job. However, with only 3 percent of the primary vote, Brown failed to get the requisite attention to be a viable contender. Kennedy's challenge attracted the most attention.

The Kennedy entry into the primaries was certain to weaken Carter's efforts for party unity. After the failed rescue attempt in Iran, the president abandoned his "rose garden" strategy and came out to contest Kennedy on April 30. President Carter took 20 of the 26 primaries where his and Kennedy's name were both listed on the ballot and proceeded to win 22 primaries to Kennedy's nine. Yet the split in the Democratic Party ultimately hurt its candidate against the unified Republicans.

THE REPUBLICAN NATIONAL CONVENTION, DETROIT, MICHIGAN, JUNE 14 TO JUNE 17

The theme of the convention was "Together...A New Beginning." The party nominated Ronald Reagan. Conventions continued to confirm candidates already determined through the caucuses and primaries. For a while it looked as if former President Gerald Ford might accept the vice-presidential spot on the ticket in a quasi co-president arrangement, but the negotiations fell through and the convention named George Bush to run for vice president. Bush, Reagan's strongest opponent in the primaries, balanced the ticket geographically. He had a home in Maine, his father had been a senator from Connecticut and his official residence was in Texas.

Representative John Anderson was introduced as a third choice in the election campaign when he announced his run for the presidency in April. Republican Anderson ran as an independent and chose former Democratic governor of Wisconsin, Patrick J. Lucey, to be his running mate. Anderson handed out 350 position papers delineating his platform and called his effort, the "National Unity Campaign."

Anderson's 15 percent standing in the polls earned him a spot in a September 21 debate televised from Baltimore, Maryland, and sponsored by the League of Women Voters. Carter declined to participate in a three-way contest, leaving Anderson and Reagan to debate. In the final election results, President Carter probably lost more votes to Anderson than Reagan did. Even though he was a lifelong Republican, Anderson's ideology seemed to be closer to his Democratic opponent. Ronald Reagan's campaign to "get government off our backs" appealed to a broad cross section of voters. The disenchanted Democrats who voted for the former California governor became known as "Reagan Democrats."

As with other incumbent presidents who have been in some political peril, Carter tried a "rose garden" strategy. The idea was to keep him focused on presidential activities and isolated from the clashes of the campaign trail. But as the 1980 canvass progressed and he was still thought to be running behind his opponent, the president could not afford to stay in the rose garden any longer. He finally agreed to debate the main contender, Ronald Reagan, but would not include John Anderson. Jimmy Carter and Ronald Reagan debated October 28 in Cleveland, Ohio. In the interchange, Reagan dismissed Carter with, "There you go again." Carter, as an evidentiary anecdote about disarmament, used a discussion with his teenage daughter Amy. Reagan, proving to his supporters his reputation as "the great communicator," closed with a series of rhetorical questions that evoked the subject of the ailing economy without allowing for a Carter response: Are you better off than you were four years ago? Is it easier for you to go and buy things in the stores? Is there more or less unemployment?

The taking of the hostages in Iran and their continued confinement took its toll on the president's re-election chances. Carter's support eroded as the days of captivity were counted down nightly before a nationwide television audience on an ABC program called "America Held Hostage." The program, specifically created to record and discuss the hostages' captivity, evolved to become ABC's "Nightline."

TELEVISION AND THE 1980 ELECTION

By 1980, the major networks were spending about $40 million and employing 1,800 people to cover the conventions. The growing costs made it even more important for the networks to attract large audiences. Though those interested in a full visual record wanted complete coverage, some in the media believed making the convention attractive to more viewers required the selective use of controversy, compelling visuals, many interviews and much commentary. Others believed that the convention news might actually be shaped by such coverage, including the "action interviews" devised to keep the convention report moving.

Presidential debates now attracted a larger television audience to the campaign than did other political events. The October 28 Reagan-

Carter debate reportedly drew in excess of 70 million viewers just a week before the November 4 election. A post-debate Gallup Poll showed a 10-plus point drop for Carter in the last two days of the campaign, the largest such change the polling organization had ever observed in a presidential election. Carter did not have time to recover after the debate.

The world of mass media, however, was about to change. The entrance of cable would diversify the industry bringing television viewers many more options and removing control of programming by only a few networks.

As 1980 dawned, the nascent Cable News Network (CNN) and the Cable Satellite Public Affairs Network (C-SPAN) began covering parts of the campaign. C-SPAN's early telecasts used video from other news sources and added its own "video verite" election coverage. Although not yet widely distributed, C-SPAN aided general understanding of the political process by covering speeches, conferences and "behind the scenes" activities. The expanded focus of political news as public affairs as introduced by CNN and C-SPAN eventually led to qualitatively different coverage of campaigns.

C-SPAN's idea of what television could be was innovative. The new cable network, which began telecasting in 1979, focused specifically on public affairs and covered events from beginning to end, "gavel to gavel," with no commercials and with no commentary from C-SPAN. As the decade progressed, candidates would have more outlets for their messages, and viewers could choose to watch entire events as well as edited portions of them.

With the emerging importance of primaries and with so many contests scheduled in so few days, "retail campaigning," where canvassing was conducted person to person and hand to hand, declined and candidates directed their strategies to increased camera coverage. By 1980, campaign managers were hiring even more media consultants, poll-takers and fundraisers to run the campaigns, further supplanting the traditional apparatus of the political parties and campaign volunteers.

◆◆◆

THE RESULTS

President Carter became the first incumbent president defeated for re-election since Herbert Hoover lost to Franklin Roosevelt in 1932. The 1980 election was the first in which women voters outnumbered men voters. Women cast more ballots for Reagan, but black voters gave him less than 10 percent. Ronald Reagan, at 69, became the oldest American president.

John Anderson illustrated the possible drawing power of an independent candidacy, at least in popular votes. He won 5,720,060 individual votes, but because he carried no state he received no votes in the Electoral College. Carter won only one state on the continent west of the Mississippi River and that was Mondale's home state of Minnesota.

Like Roosevelt, Reagan brought others of his party with him to Washington. The Republicans, with 12 new members, gained control of the Senate, 53 seats to 47 seats, and made some progress in the House of Representatives where the Democrats lost 33 seats and the seat count became 243 Democrats to 192 Republicans.

1980

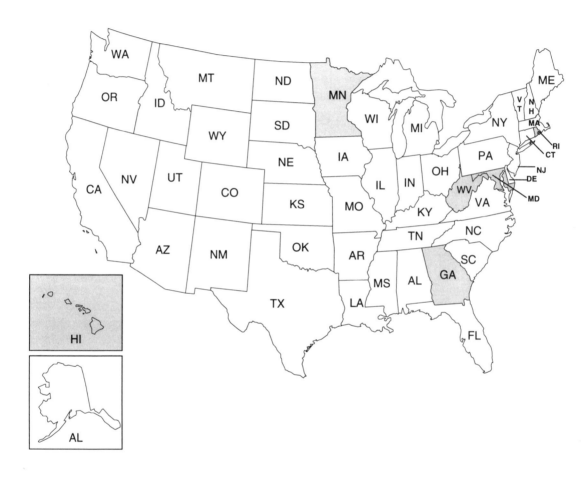

☐ Reagan (Republican)

▨ Carter (Democrat)

POSTSCRIPT

The international crisis that had so bedeviled Jimmy Carter's last year in office was nonexistent for Ronald Reagan. On Inauguration Day, the 52 remaining American hostages were freed from Iranian control. The new president was able to announce to the world that the Americans were on their way back home. Network coverage of the release was juxtaposed with live coverage of Reagan's inauguration ceremony.

On March 30, 1981, Ronald Reagan was shot and wounded outside the Washington Hilton Hotel and became the first president to be hit by an assassin's bullet and survive. Reagan, although more seriously wounded than first thought, maintained his sense of humor at the hospital: "I hope you're all Republicans," he quipped.

During his first administration, Reagan implemented the tax cut of 1981, appointed Sandra Day O'Connor as the first woman justice on the U.S. Supreme Court, presided over a deep recession in 1982, sent American troops to Grenada and Lebanon and extended unemployment benefits to those left jobless by the recession.

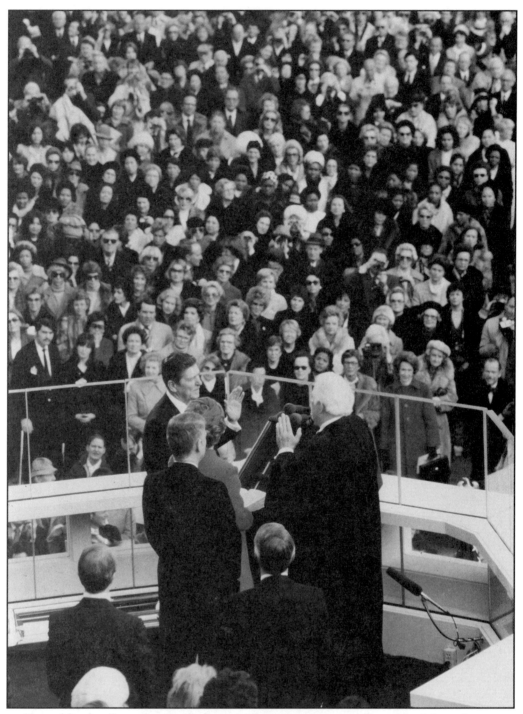

Upon his election at age 69, Ronald Reagan became the oldest American president. *(C-SPAN photo.)*

"So, as we begin, let us take inventory. We are a nation that has a government—not the other way around. And this makes us special among the nations of the Earth. Our Government has no power except that granted it by the people. It is time to check and reverse the growth of government which shows signs of having grown beyond the consent of the governed.

It is my intention to curb the size and influence of the Federal establishment and to demand recognition of the distinction between the powers granted to the Federal Government and those reserved to the States or to the people. All of us need to be reminded that the Federal Government did not create the States; the States created the Federal Government.

Now, so there will be no misunderstanding, it is not my intention to do away with government. It is, rather, to make it work—work with us, not over us; to stand by our side, not ride on our back. Government can and must provide opportunity, not smother it; foster productivity, not stifle it."

President Ronald Reagan
Inaugural Address
January 20, 1981

== 10 ==

THE ELECTION OF 1984

*Population of the United States: **236.35 million***
*Number of eligible voters: **174.47 million***
*Percent of those eligible who voted: **53.1***
*Percent of television saturation in U.S. households: **98***

SETTING THE STAGE

A merica is back—standing tall, looking to the eighties with courage, confidence, and hope," said President Reagan in the State of the Union address on January 25, 1981. But in the same speech, he blunted the optimism when he called on Congress to help cut the budget deficit by more than $100 billion over the succeeding three years.

The fiscal difficulties inherent in federal government spending provided ample reason to call for austerity. Budget deficits were at record levels and the national debt was proliferating even though the economy had grown at 6.8 percent and personal income had also risen. There were other signs of problems ahead. Over 80 savings and loan associations were near insolvency, and their eventual demise marked the largest failure of U.S. financial institutions since the late 1930s. Further, 1984 saw a record trade deficit. The inflation rate was down to about 4 percent for the year, but the unemployment rate hovered just above 7 percent. The average cost to purchase a new single-family home was a record $101,000. An optimist had plenty to crow about and a pessimist had evidence to forecast gloom and doom. It was a confusing mix of economic news.

The demographic trends of the last presidential elections continued. The South and West gained residents while population in the Northeast and the Midwest stayed about the same. Seven states each had more than a million residents over age 65. Both the geographical shift and the rising population of older voters would continue to affect the political landscape.

International events were also causing concern at home. There was considerable controversy in April 1984 when Congress learned that the CIA had mined the harbors of Nicaragua two months earlier. Later in April, President Reagan withdrew the remaining U.S. Marines from Beirut, Lebanon. This followed the October 23, 1983, suicide bombing that killed 241 Marines in their barracks. The Marines had been in Lebanon off and on since peacekeeping forces were sent in August of 1982.

◆◆◆

THE CANDIDATES AND THE ISSUES

PRESIDENT RONALD REAGAN, THE REPUBLICAN PARTY CANDIDATE
(Ronald Reagan's biography is in chapter nine.)

FORMER VICE PRESIDENT WALTER F. MONDALE,
THE DEMOCRATIC PARTY CANDIDATE

Mondale was born on January 5, 1928, in Ceylon, Minnesota. He attended Macalester College and graduated from the University of Minnesota in 1951. After serving in the Army during the Korean War, Mondale earned a law degree from the University of Minnesota law school in 1956.

Mondale was active in Minnesota's Democratic Farmer-Labor Party and was appointed assistant to the state's attorney general in 1958. In 1960, he was appointed to the attorney general's unexpired term and won election in his own right for that post in the same year. He was re-elected in 1962. In 1964, Mondale was appointed to finish the Senate term of Democrat Hubert Humphrey when Humphrey was elected vice president under President Johnson. Mondale won his own Senate term in 1966 and was re-elected in 1972.

In 1976, Mondale was elected vice president of the United States on the Jimmy Carter ticket. President Carter and Vice President

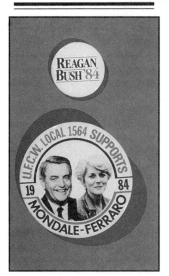

(Campaign materials courtesy private collection of Dr. John Sullivan, University of Virginia/Photo by Paul Kennedy.)

Mondale lost their re-election bid in 1980. After his defeat in the 1984 election, Mondale returned to the private practice of law. In 1993 he was named U.S. Ambassador to Japan under the Clinton administration.

◆◆◆

THE ISSUES

President Reagan campaigned by emphasizing a growing U.S. economy and general peace around the world. Knowing that overall peace and prosperity was a tough combination to run against, the Democrats attempted to counter Reagan's campaign message. They emphasized the negative economic indicators, especially the shrinking American job base.

Former Vice President Mondale was more of a New Deal Democrat than President Carter had been. Facing an uphill race against Reagan, Mondale and his team knew they had to campaign with new ideas and take risks. Mondale ventured big when he said he would raise taxes if elected president, an unusual statement in a national election. He also asserted that Reagan would raise taxes too but would not admit that to the American people.

RONALD REAGAN, REPUBLICAN

The president campaigned on a platform of controlling the size of the federal government. He advocated reducing government spending, holding the line on taxes, passing a tuition tax credit and reforming the federal tax system to yield a fair and simple tax. He opposed "protectionist" tariffs. Reagan favored a line-item veto and wanted to pass two constitutional amendments: one to ban abortions and another to balance the federal budget.

Reagan supported strong military preparedness. He backed protection of human rights as "the moral center of our foreign policy." The president insisted on supporting efforts to achieve democracy in Central America, and wanted to continue negotiating arms control with the Soviet Union and upgrade "hotline communications" with Moscow.

WALTER MONDALE, DEMOCRAT

Mondale told the American people it would be necessary to raise taxes to reduce deficit spending. He supported enforcement of civil rights laws and was committed to affirmative action efforts. The former vice president urged preservation of the environment and supported passage of the equal rights amendment. He opposed a constitutional amendment to ban abortion.

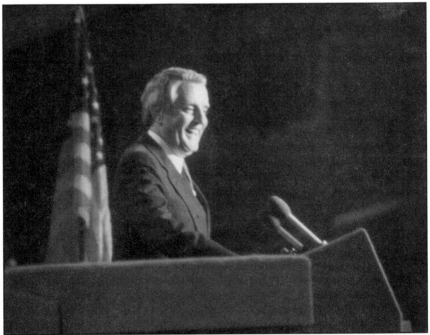

Former Vice President Walter Mondale won the Democratic presidential nomination in 1984. His vice-presidential running mate, Geraldine Ferraro, was the first woman to appear on a majority-party ticket.
(Credit: Consolidated News Pictures/Photo by Ron Sachs.)

Mondale called for a strong defense, but opposed construction of the B-1 bomber, the MX missile and the Reagan administration's SDI, a space-based defense system which he said would turn "the heavens into a battleground." Mondale advocated annual summit meetings with the Soviet Union and international negotiations for arms control along with a "nuclear freeze."

THE CAMPAIGN

During the Iowa caucuses, former Vice President Mondale came out ahead, winning 46 percent of the Democratic support. This represented a significant lead over his competitors, Senator Gary Hart of Colorado with 16 percent and Senator George McGovern with 13 percent. Gary Hart surprised observers by his showing ahead of McGovern in Iowa. With the momentum, Hart proceeded to win the New Hampshire primary, 39 percent to 29 percent over Mondale, and made a sweep of northern New England with victories in Maine and Vermont. The young senator's offer of "new ideas for a new generation of Americans" struck a responsive chord with the electorate.

On Super Tuesday, March 13, Hart was victorious in Florida, Massachusetts and Rhode Island. Mondale won Illinois on March 20 and then won New York with 45 percent of the votes to Hart's 27 percent. The Reverend Jesse Jackson was close to Hart in New York with 26 percent of the votes. After Mondale won the Pennsylvania contest on April 10, Jackson won in the District of Columbia with two-thirds of the votes. Mondale, Jackson and Hart then split Tennessee, Louisiana and Indiana respectively.

THE DEMOCRATIC CONVENTION, SAN FRANCISCO, CALIFORNIA, JULY 16 TO JULY 19

At the end of the primary season, Hart had won 14 primaries, Mondale 11 and Jackson two. However, Walter Mondale went to the Democratic convention with the majority of committed delegates behind him. The strong challenge of Gary Hart had fallen short. Mondale's long-standing service to the party brought him the support of party regulars and sufficient additional delegates to boost him over Hart and Jackson at the convention.

As the presidential candidate, Mondale then chose his running mate, Geraldine Ferraro, a three-term member of Congress from New York. This was the first time a woman had received a nomination on a major-party ticket. Jesse Jackson and New York Governor Mario Cuomo both gave well-received speeches. The boldest statement came from Mondale's acceptance speech and would provoke headlines and discussion throughout the campaign: "Mr. Reagan will raise taxes, and so will I. He won't tell you. I just did."

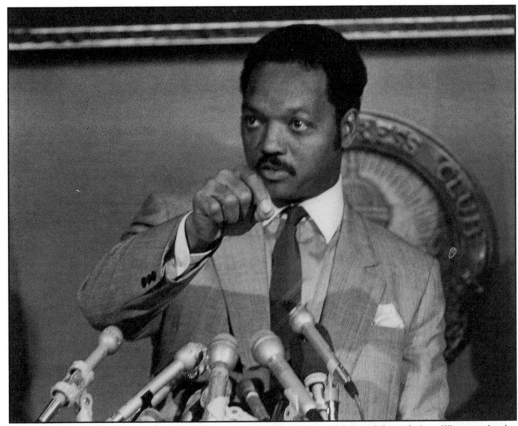

Going into the Democratic National Convention, Walter Mondale still needed delegates to boost him over Senator Gary Hart and the Reverend Jesse Jackson for the nomination. *(C-SPAN photo.)*

Reagan won 86 percent of the vote in the Republican primary in New Hampshire on February 28. His campaign moved without challenge to a renomination by acclamation at the convention. It was the first time Republicans had used only a single roll-call vote to select both nominees. The ticket was again Ronald Reagan and George Bush.

Televised debates were now expected in the presidential campaigns. Even incumbents like Reagan were pressured by the public to face their opponents in debate. The 1984 presidential candidates met for two televised debates. On October 7, when President Reagan and former Vice President Mondale met in the Kentucky Center for the Arts auditorium in Louisville, the discussion centered on taxes and the national debt. Some political observers believed that Mondale held his own with the president and some felt he had surpassed the incumbent in the cogency of his arguments. At times some of the press noted that Reagan seemed unsteady and unsure of his answers, raising questions about his age.

The candidates met once again in Kansas City, Missouri, on October 21. Reagan preempted any questions about his age by saying, "I am not going to exploit for political purposes, my opponent's youth and inexperience." After the exchange, age ceased being an issue in the campaign and other concerns about Reagan's leadership seemed to fade away as well.

The vice-presidential nominees debated from a studio in Philadelphia, Pennsylvania, on October 11. After the confrontation, Geraldine Ferraro charged George Bush with being "patronizing."

In the contemporary media campaign, personal controversy attracts an audience and frequents the nightly news. This was especially apparent when questions about the finances of Ferraro's husband became part of the campaign story. It was also news when New York's Roman Catholic Archbishop, John J. O'Connor, attacked Representative Ferraro, a Catholic, for what he saw as her permissive position on abortion. Democrats argued that the personal issues were tangential at best, but Ferraro's problems diverted the Democratic candidates from the substantive issues that they thought would constitute their trump card in the campaign.

President Reagan began his final canvass "to make America great again" in his home state of California. Geraldine Ferraro spoke in California toward the end of her campaign. Her appearance, in San Francisco, was announced as "A Moment in History."

Television and the 1984 Campaign

As the 1984 election approached, the major networks looked at revenues and the number of viewers who tuned in to political conventions. They saw that independent stations and even some network affiliates were choosing more lucrative entertainment programming over the convention coverage. The viewing audience in general was also being pulled away from the broadcast networks by the growing number of choices on cable television. The broadcast hegemony was beginning to yield to a more competitive television environment. For ABC, CBS and NBC, keeping the audience meant changing the way elections were covered. They moved to crisper commentary, an accent on controversy and an expanded focus on personality.

Even with this splintering of the viewing audience, the diversification of cable options actually served to increase coverage of campaigns overall. Two in particular, the Cable Satellite Public Affairs Network (C-SPAN) and the Cable News Network (CNN) had established their own niches: CNN's all-news format put more political news on the air, and C-SPAN ventured into the field with its no-commentary format and gavel-to-gavel coverage. Available in 16 million homes, C-SPAN covered the Iowa caucuses in 1984, the first time a network had telecast an entire caucus, gavel to gavel. C-SPAN cameras went "live" to a caucus of 15 in the home of a hog farmer and a caucus of 100 at a downtown Des Moines high school. Even some residents of Iowa had never seen what went on inside their celebrated political meetings. C-SPAN continued its long-form video coverage of the campaign with a "grass-roots" crew riding in a Winnebago to study the election process in 14 cities around the United States.

It was at the national conventions that the new type of coverage offered by the cable networks began to noticeably bifurcate from that of the broadcast networks. Just as the networks were limiting their political coverage, C-SPAN and CNN were expanding theirs. The Public Broadcasting Service (PBS) also provided extensive coverage to its member stations.

From the early announcements through the final whirlwind tour, television was now an integral part of the political process. Ronald Reagan, the former actor, had the requisite skills for this new era of media saturation, whereas Walter Mondale appeared less comfortable with it. Reagan was to television what Franklin D. Roosevelt had been to radio. Using the dominant medium of their time, each communicated adroitly with the public. The Republicans used television strategically. Even before the campaign began in earnest, the administration had prepared a "message of the day" technique to help shape what was shown on the nightly news; they also worked to provide producers with stimulating visuals.

By 1984, politics had become an industry, employing professional managers, computer-savvy staffs, pollsters, media consultants and expert advance workers. Both those behind the cameras and those in front of them operated under great pressure. Miscues on either end, beamed instantly across the nation, could alter the outcome of an election.

Political advertising had become an art form unto itself. The Republicans' group of professional communicators known as the "Tuesday Team" created commercials for the president with wholesome images. Their signature commercial was an 18-minute Reagan biography called "Morning in America," with segments to run also in 30-second to five-minute spots. Tracking polls indicating the ad campaign was working signaled the continuing significance of television commercials for all candidates. Collecting large sums of money to fund presidential campaigns took on great importance. Expensive advertising agencies and prime time spots on television cost candidates millions of dollars in 1984.

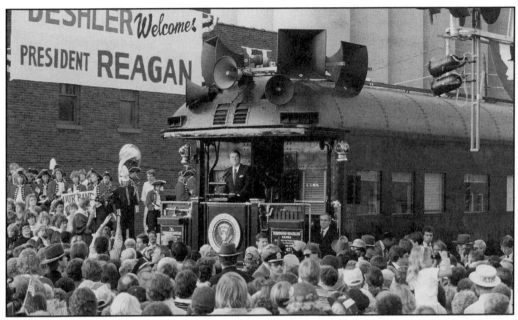

Ronald Reagan, as a former actor, was comfortable with television and the media, and used his skills to communicate his message to the public. *(Courtesy Ronald Reagan Library.)*

THE RESULTS

An incumbent running on peace and prosperity, especially when slogan and reality seem in tandem, has been hard to beat at any time in American history. President Reagan's personal popularity added to the general perception of well-being in the country and made him unbeatable. Democratic Speaker of the House Thomas "Tip" O'Neill spoke to the president's political strength when he said, "Reagan is the most popular figure in the history of the United States. No candidate we put up would have beat Reagan this year." And Lloyd Bentsen, Democratic senator from Texas, said of George Bush, "The only test of

1984

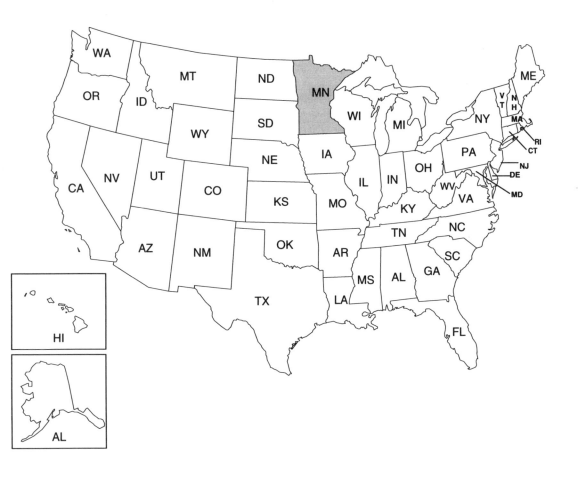

☐ Reagan (Republican)

▨ Mondale (Democrat)

a good vice president is loyalty to the president. By that test, George Bush has done an excellent job."

President Reagan won the majority of votes from every age group. He carried Catholic voters by 61 percent to 39 percent and women by 55 percent to 45 percent. Mondale prevailed among black voters and members of unions. Mondale's 52 percent support from union voters was considerably less than past Democratic candidates. Reagan's landslide included the support of a majority of people under age 24. The youth vote and his share of women voters moved both of these demographic groups into the Republican column. Prior to 1980, they had been more likely to vote for Democratic candidates.

Reagan almost won all 50 states, losing only Mondale's home state of Minnesota by 0.2 of a percentage point. Mondale also won in the District of Columbia. Only Richard Nixon in 1972 had previously been victorious in 49 states. Ronald Reagan also won a record 525 electoral votes.

In his book of collected speeches, *Speaking My Mind*, Reagan wrote: "The story of 1984 is the election. The economy was humming, the world was fairly quiet, the wheels of government were turning so the nation and the media focused on politics."

POSTSCRIPT

President Reagan's second inaugural took place on a day so cold that as the temperature dropped to 9 degrees the ceremony was moved inside to the Capitol Rotunda.

Early in his first administration, President Reagan had delivered some strong words to the Soviet Union and relations continued to be strained. By the end of his second term, however, the two countries had improved communication and begun positive discussions on arms control. In addition to the somewhat tough negotiations with the Soviets, the administration had eventful clashes with Iran, Libya and Nicaragua. In 1985, Reagan agreed to impose sanctions against South

Africa. He vetoed a more stringent bill in 1986, but Congress overrode the veto and the bill became law.

The home front saw general prosperity, yet Reagan presided over the highest federal budget deficits in American history. He tried to mitigate the problem by signing into law a 1986 overhaul of the tax system and the Gramm-Rudman-Hollings Act, which aimed toward a balanced budget. He became the first president to submit a trillion dollar budget to Congress.

"The time has come for a new American emancipation—a great national drive to tear down economic barriers and liberate the spirit of enterprise in the most distressed areas of our country. My friends, together we can do this, and do it we must, so help me God.

From new freedom will spring new opportunities for growth, a more productive, fulfilled and united people and a strong America—an America that will lead the technological revolution, and also open its mind and heart and soul to the treasures of literature, music, and poetry, and the values of faith, courage, and love."

President Ronald Reagan
Second Inaugural Address
January 21, 1985

= 11 =
THE ELECTION OF 1988

*Population of the United States: **245.02 million***
*Number of eligible voters: **182.78 million***
*Percent of those eligible who voted: **50.1***
*Percent of television saturation in U.S. households: **98***

SETTING THE STAGE

In 1988, as the baby boom generation grew older, the American population was no longer characterized by youth. In fact, the median age of Americans was over 32 years old for the first time in history. Rural citizens continued to migrate to more populous areas. More than half of new mothers were returning to the work force shortly after having their babies. The percentage of Americans who voted in the 1988 presidential election continued its downward slide.

Ronald Reagan was the first president since Dwight Eisenhower to complete two full terms. At the end of his second administration, most sectors of the economy were doing well. In April 1988, the unemployment rate was 5.4 percent. Inflation, however, was still high and the Federal Reserve Board raised its discount rate to 6.5 percent. Banks set their prime borrowing rate at 10 percent; the "prime" went up four times in 1988. Health care costs were also afflicting the economy as they now accounted for an estimated 11.1 percent of the gross national product.

On January 2, 1988, President Reagan and Canadian Prime Minister Brian Mulroney agreed to lower trade barriers between their two countries. On February 5, federal grand juries in Miami and Tampa indicted Panama's leader General Manuel Antonio Noriega on charges of bribery and narcotics trafficking. After occupying Afghanistan for nine years, the Soviet Union began pulling out its troops on April 14, 1988. The Soviets and the Americans would subsequently co-sponsor a Smithsonian Institution exhibit, "Crossroads of Siberia and Alaska," the first significant cultural exchange between the two world powers since the start of the Cold War. The French re-elected President Francois Mitterand on July 8, over Jacques Chirac. Benazir Bhutto was elected Prime Minister of Pakistan. And, on August 8, after eight years of fighting, Iraq and Iran agreed to a truce.

Beginning in the summer of 1987, a political controversy was played out to an American television audience. Marine Lieutenant Colonel Oliver North gave dramatic testimony before a congressional committee concerning allegations of selling arms to Iran and using the funds to support insurgents in Nicaragua. The testimony of North, a National Security Council aide said to be involved in the dealings, was seen by a television audience of millions. During the course of the hearings, links between what became known as "Iran-Contra" and Vice President Bush were implied, but no connection was proved. President Reagan cited reasons of national security and executive privilege in order to withhold certain government documents requested for North's defense. On March 16, 1988, a federal grand jury handed down 14 indictments in the case.

THE CANDIDATES AND THE ISSUES

VICE PRESIDENT GEORGE HERBERT WALKER BUSH, THE REPUBLICAN PARTY CANDIDATE

Bush was born at his family's home in Milton, Massachusetts on June 12, 1924. He married Barbara Pierce on January 6, 1945. They had two daughters, Robin and Dorothy, and four sons, George W., John "Jeb," Neil and Marvin. George and Barbara Bush divided their time between a home in Texas and a summer residence in Kennebunkport, Maine.

As the son of U.S. Senator Prescott Bush of Connecticut, George Bush grew up around politics.

George Bush joined the Navy during World War II, became a combat pilot in the Pacific and rose to the rank of lieutenant. He graduated in 1948 from Yale University. Bush was co-founder of Zapata Offshore Company, an oil and gas business, and later became its president.

In 1964, Bush lost the election for a U.S. Senate seat from Texas, but won a seat in the House of Representatives in 1966. He was in the House from 1967 to 1971, and lost in another bid for the Senate in 1970. He was then appointed to be the Permanent Representative of the United States to the United Nations, serving from 1971 to 1972. In 1973, President Nixon appointed Bush as chairman of the Republican National Committee. He left this position when Nixon resigned the presidency in 1974. President Ford then appointed Bush to be U.S. Liaison Officer in China. In 1976, Ford appointed him to be the director of the CIA, a post he held from 1976 to 1977. In 1980, Bush was elected vice president on Ronald Reagan's ticket. He served for two terms, 1981 to 1989, and was known for his loyalty to the president.

After serving one term as president, Bush lost his bid for re-election and retired in 1992.

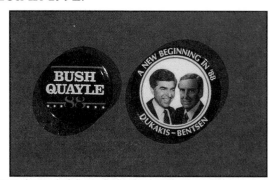

(Campaign materials courtesy private collection of Dr. John Sullivan, University of Virginia/Photo by Paul Kennedy.)

MASSACHUSETTS GOVERNOR MICHAEL S. DUKAKIS, THE DEMOCRATIC PARTY CANDIDATE

Dukakis was born November 3, 1933, in Brookline, Massachusetts. He graduated from Swarthmore College in 1955 and Harvard law school in 1960. He served in the Army during the Korean war.

In 1962, he was elected to the Massachusetts State Legislature and served from 1963 until 1971. In 1970, he was defeated in an election for lieutenant governor of Massachusetts. He was the moderator from 1971 to 1973 for "The Advocates," a public television show that debated public policy issues. Dukakis won his first term as governor of Massachusetts in 1974, but lost his party's nomination in 1978. From 1978 to 1982, he taught at the Kennedy School of Government at Harvard. He won the governorship again in 1982 and 1986.

After the 1988 presidential election, Dukakis returned to teaching and continued to speak on public issues.

THE ISSUES

The Republicans had controlled the executive office for eight years. Nominee George Bush was not as popular as Ronald Reagan, but Bush had been waiting in the wings and was willing to pursue many of the Reagan policies. He also had over 20 years of public service, including time as the chairman of the Republican National Committee. In the campaign, Bush argued that his experience in international affairs distinguished him from his opponent, Governor Michael Dukakis. Dukakis emphasized domestic issues and his intention to bring the "Massachusetts Miracle" of a revitalized economy to the whole country.

Although the campaign turned out to be a vigorous one, neither candidate called for radical change. Bush wanted to preserve the prosperity from previous Republican administrations, and Dukakis wanted to pursue traditional Democratic programs by making them more efficient.

GEORGE BUSH, REPUBLICAN
The vice president campaigned on the promise to promote the Reagan agenda. He called for a strong America in order to maintain peace and put forth a "no new taxes" promise to keep the economy prosperous. He wanted to reduce the capital gains tax and instigate a system of tax credits that could be used by families for child care. He called for a constitutional amendment to require a balanced budget.

Bush wanted a line-item veto power for the president and he favored congressional term limits. He campaigned strongly for crime prevention efforts and favored the death penalty. Bush also ran against "liberals," whom he blamed for excessive regulation that had hindered business growth. Bush took a strong stand against abortion, calling it an example of the "permissive liberal culture" of the late 1980s.

The vice president emphasized patriotism and advocated building a strong defense and a space-based defense shield.

Michael Dukakis, Democrat

The Massachusetts governor maintained that the campaign was about competence and that he would bring competence to Washington. He called for a more efficient yet compassionate government. He believed that cutting the deficit was necessary for the country's future prosperity. He endorsed establishing more child care centers and advocated an employer-financed national health insurance program. Dukakis opposed the death penalty and supported a woman's "right to choose" on abortion. He condemned the "sleaze" in the Republican administration.

The Democratic candidate wanted to maintain a strong America but advocated spending more money on a high-speed, conventional military than on expensive, experimental and highly technological defense systems.

◆◆◆

The Campaign

The 1988 election was a spirited one. Both parties knew they had a good chance at winning this contest. The Democrats would not have to face the popular Ronald Reagan, who could not seek a third term under the provisions of the 22nd Amendment; and the Republicans had a full field of possible candidates. Among the Republican candidates who wanted the nomination were Vice President George Bush, former Secretary of State Alexander Haig, Representative Jack Kemp of New York, the Reverend Pat Robertson and Senate Minority Leader Robert Dole of Kansas.

Bob Dole won the Iowa caucuses with 37.4 percent of the vote to Pat Robertson's 24.6 percent and Bush's 18.6 percent. But Bush was able to outmatch Dole in the media-saturated primary in New Hampshire, a state close in proximity to Bush's base of support in Maine. Bush garnered 37.6 percent of the vote; whereas Dole won 28.4 percent. Pat Robertson finished a distant fourth. The recharged Bush campaign won all of the primaries on Super Tuesday.

The Democrats also had several candidates vying for the nomination. Former Senator Gary Hart of Colorado and the Reverend Jesse Jackson were back from the 1984 race. The others were Massachusetts Governor Michael Dukakis, Tennessee Senator Albert Gore Jr., Illinois Senator Paul Simon, Missouri Representative Richard Gephardt, former Arizona Governor Bruce Babbitt and Delaware Senator Joseph Biden.

Early in the race, it looked as if Gary Hart would be the front-runner, but he dropped out in May 1987 after the Miami Herald reported his relationship with a woman who was not his wife.

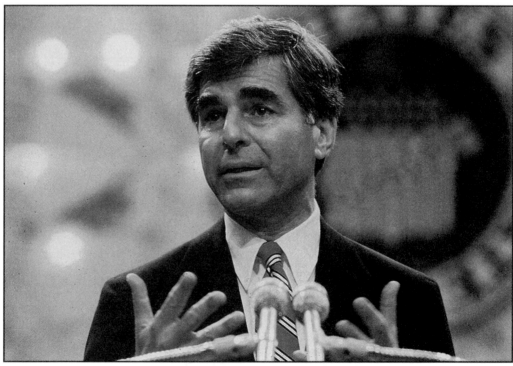

In his campaign, Massachusetts Governor Michael Dukakis stated he would bring the "Massachusetts Miracle" of a revitalized economy to the whole country. *(Credit: Consolidated News Pictures/Photo by Ron Sachs.)*

Joseph Biden abandoned his effort in the fall of 1987, after charges that he plagiarized parts of speeches of a British politician and misstated his academic record. This trend toward public discussion of personal peccadillos continued, raising issues of media ethics and responsibility in reporting. Increased media attention sometimes moved the focus of campaigns away from issues of substance and towards peripheral issues.

The prizes in the primary season were the votes of hundreds of delegates from 38 primaries and caucuses. Governor Dukakis started poorly, finishing third in the Iowa caucuses behind Gephardt and Simon. He made a significant comeback on February 16, winning in his neighboring state of New Hampshire. This was succeeded by an impressive showing on Super Tuesday, when Dukakis won seven out of the 19 primaries on that day. Because he was better funded than the other candidates at this stage, he was able to buy more targeted television time. Jesse Jackson won the March 26 Michigan primary, 55 percent to Dukakis's 28 percent. Dukakis won in New York on April 19, defeating both Jackson and Al Gore, and won in Pennsylvania over Jackson the next week, 67 percent to 27 percent. On June 7, Dukakis won California, Montana, New Jersey and New Mexico and it was all over.

THE DEMOCRATIC NATIONAL CONVENTION, ATLANTA, GEORGIA, JULY 18 TO JULY 21

Jesse Jackson, seeking the nomination for a second time, pursued it right up to the convention even though he was well behind in the delegate count. On the first ballot, the convention confirmed Dukakis of Massachusetts as the party's presidential nominee and Senator Lloyd Bentsen of Texas as their vice-presidential nominee. The ticket replicated the geographic balance of the winning 1960 Democratic ticket: John F. Kennedy from Massachusetts and Lyndon Johnson from Texas. Dukakis established the theme of his candidacy in his acceptance speech when he said that the campaign was "not about ideology. It's about competence."

**THE REPUBLICAN NATIONAL CONVENTION,
NEW ORLEANS, LOUISIANA, AUGUST 15 TO AUGUST 18**
Bush's victories in the primaries and caucuses led to a first ballot nomination at the convention. At an outdoor rally in the Spanish Plaza, he announced his choice for a running mate, J. Danforth "Dan" Quayle, a 41-year-old senator from Indiana. Quayle contributed a base in a Midwestern state to the ticket and a connection to younger voters.

In his acceptance speech, Bush promised that he would not recommend any new taxes. "Read my lips," he stated. "No new taxes." It was a pledge that would be quoted back to him many times late in his administration, when he agreed to an increase in taxes. He also called for "a kinder gentler nation."

From the very beginning of the race, Bush's campaign team attacked Dukakis and Democratic policies. Alleging that Democratic positions on the death penalty and prison furloughs showed a "softness" on crime, the Republicans arranged for the Boston Police Patrolman's Association to appear behind Bush for a September 22 photo opportunity in front of the television cameras. In addition, they ridiculed Dukakis's stance as an environmentalist in a television commercial reportedly showing a polluted Boston Harbor. As governor, Dukakis had opposed a mandatory recitation of the Pledge of Allegiance in the Massachusetts schools. Bush labeled this stand permissive and suggested that if Dukakis were elected he might expand his "liberal" agenda to the whole nation. The vice president repeated the label "liberal" as if it were a slander yet little rebuttal came from Dukakis. If Dukakis would not define himself in the election, Bush would do it for him. Bush characterized himself as the steward of the Reagan tradition.

According to most prognosticators, Dukakis emerged from the Democratic convention in the lead. But even after seeing his reputed advantage narrow shortly after the Republican convention, Dukakis failed to reignite his campaign until after Labor Day, when the contest was drawing near. Once it was clear that Bush was surging in the polls, the Dukakis campaign did accelerate. The Democrats committed some blunders, however. In trying to win over constituencies who wanted a stronger military, Dukakis was shown on television riding in a tank, but wearing an oversized helmet. The Republicans made a commercial ridiculing the image. In addition, Dukakis failed to respond to Republican commercials that alleged he was soft on crime.

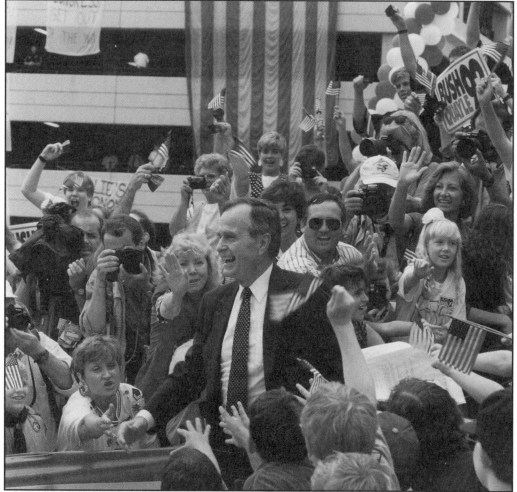

Upon winning the 1988 election, George Bush became the first sitting vice president to be elected president since Martin Van Buren in 1836. *(Courtesy Bush Presidential Materials Project.)*

The first presidential debate aired September 25 from Wake Forest University in North Carolina and most pundits scored it a draw. In the second debate, however, the opening question underscored a perceived Dukakis weakness. The governor appeared to be caught off guard when CNN's Bernard Shaw asked a hypothetical question about what his response would be to an attack on his wife. Dukakis's answer was specific enough, as he restated his position on crime and the death penalty, but his response, to a clearly poignant situation, lacked any visible emotion. Shortly after this debate, polls showed Dukakis behind by over 10 percentage points.

Unlike Carter in 1980, who had lost momentum in the waning hours of that campaign, Dukakis made a final advance at the end. Efforts to lighten his image and make him appear more personable seemed to be working, but it was not enough to threaten Bush. Dukakis's popularity had gone down during the course of the campaign, but the popularity of his running mate, Lloyd Bentsen, went up. Bentsen seemed to get the best of the Republican nominee, Dan Quayle, in their vice-presidential debate, and to some Bentsen seemed to be more presidential than Dukakis.

Television and the 1988 Campaign

Public affairs cable television continued to expand and grow. In this election year, C-SPAN, at almost 10 years old, had established itself as the network of record for covering the major-party conventions from gavel to gavel without interruption. The network also covered the caucuses, the primaries and the campaign. Its "Road to the White House" series sought to bring the whole electoral process to the voter and began its coverage as soon as the earliest exploratory candidates went to Iowa and New Hampshire.

CNN was also heavily involved in campaign coverage, and the broadcast networks continued to cover the highlights of the campaign on their nightly news programs. CNN's daily "Inside Politics" became a staple for many who could not get enough political information elsewhere.

Television continued to be a major factor in candidate selection and escalated the cost of campaigns. For example, it was impossible for candidates to canvass personally all 19 states holding primaries on Super Tuesday, and they had to be well funded to conduct a television campaign. Satellites that could now transmit campaign messages to targeted audiences—to viewers in a state hosting a primary contest perhaps—came at a price.

Television news shows favored campaign pictures of candidates that were visually stimulating. The staging of such photo opportunities was sometimes less than effective, such as Dukakis's ride in an army tank and Bush's pose in full Native American headdress. Media consultants who tried to show the candidates at their best, also limited access to the nominee to avoid negative situations. Because reporters want to get as close to candidates as possible, limiting this access often required more skill than staging media events

A network news anchor became a part of the campaign story early in 1988. During a live interview, CBS Evening News anchor Dan Rather confronted the vice president on his knowledge of diversion of funds in the reputed "Iran-Contra" connection. Bush sharply responded, "I want to talk about why I want to be president." Bush proceeded to attack the substance and mode of Rather's questioning saying, "I don't have respect for what you are doing here tonight." Bush's supporters claimed their man got the best of the encounter against a seemingly contentious newscaster.

Bush's campaign also used political advertisements effectively to fend off opponents. A Bush ad claimed that his Republican opponent Bob Dole had "straddled" on the issue of raising taxes. Shortly after the New Hampshire primary, this charge evoked an angry televised response from Dole, who warned Bush to "stop lying about my record." The incident hurt Dole and Bush scored heavily against him on Super Tuesday.

Adding to Dukakis's media woes was the Bush campaign team's effective use of television commercials right up to Election Day. The "Revolving Door" commercial implied that Dukakis supported an indiscriminate prison furlough program in Massachusetts. The ad was confused by some viewers with a negative ad prepared and sponsored by an independent group which exploited the 1986 case of Willie Horton, a convicted felon who committed violent crimes while on furlough from a Massachusetts prison. An unchallenged attack soon took on the aura of fact and the Republicans took advantage of Dukakis's lack of response. Bush had a series of positive ads as well. Called the "I Am That Man" commercials, they emphasized that the vice president could provide "Experienced Leadership for America's Future."

The Dukakis commercials probably failed to increase his final vote total. An anti-Bush ad called "The Handlers" suggested, perhaps too subtly, that Bush and Quayle were manipulated by their aides. "They'd like to sell you a package," it claimed, but "wouldn't you rather choose a president?"

Televised presidential debates were again an important feature of the campaign. Candidates feared that failure to enter the debates would appear as a sign of weakness on the issues. The televised debates also provided the opportunity to create and enhance an image, and both sides worked to shape debate coverage. Because Dukakis was much shorter than Bush, the "debate rules" required that the two debaters would appear close in height. Podiums were built to different heights and a "pitcher's mound" was built to put Dukakis in direct eye contact with the cameras.

There appeared to be a made-for-television moment in the vice-presidential debate when Dan Quayle attempted to refute suggestions that he was too young and inexperienced to be vice president. Quayle asserted that he was no younger or less experienced than John Kennedy when Kennedy was elected president. "Senator," retorted the Democratic nominee, Bentsen, "I served with Jack Kennedy. I knew Jack Kennedy. Jack Kennedy was a friend of mine. Senator, you're no Jack Kennedy." It was one of the most striking sound bites in the campaign.

THE RESULTS

In a hard-fought and frequently bitter campaign, Vice President George Bush defeated Massachusetts Governor Michael Dukakis. The voter turnout was the lowest in 64 years. Bush carried 40 states and received 426 electoral votes and 48,886,097 popular votes, or 53.4 percent of the total votes. Dukakis took 10 states plus the District of Columbia, 111 electoral votes and 41,809,074 popular votes or 45.6 percent of the total. The Republican victory, however, did not carry into Congress. The Democrats won one additional Senate seat, now holding a 55 seat to 45 seat majority. In the House, the Democrats gained three seats for a 260 seat to 175 seat majority.

George Bush was the first sitting vice president to be elected president since Martin Van Buren in 1836.

1988

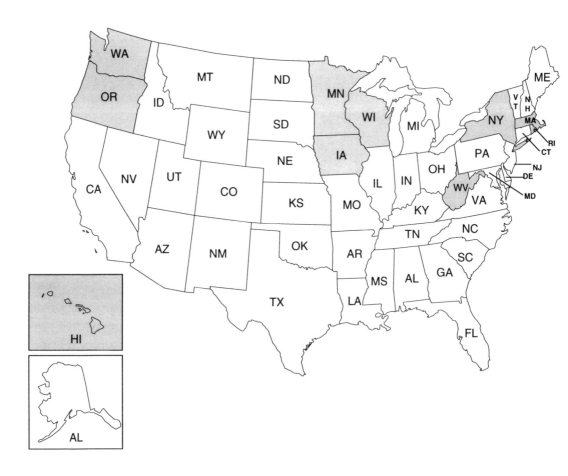

Bush (Republican)

Dukakis (Democrat)

Postscript

During President Bush's term in office, phenomenal world events unfolded as the Berlin Wall fell in 1989 and the Soviet Union dissolved into separate republics. Bush presided over a military action in Panama and successfully led American and Allied troops in an effort to quell the advances of the Iraqi army in the Middle East. Bush took a firm stand against Iraqi President Saddam Hussein and immediately dispatched U.S. troops to the Persian Gulf to halt the invasion of Kuwait by the Hussein forces.

On the home front, however, Bush broke one promise that a number of Americans were loath to forget in the next election cycle. To deal with the burgeoning deficit, he agreed to sign a tax increase and his "read my lips—no new taxes" assurance would come back to haunt him. On July 26, 1990, the president endorsed the Americans with Disabilities Act, and later in the same year signed a strengthened Clean Air Act.

The president and Barbara Bush were personally popular. Bush was thought of as most successful in international affairs. But his purported neglect of domestic affairs in the midst of high prices took its toll in the last year and a half of his term.

"My friends, we are not the sum of our possessions. They are not the measure of our lives. In our hearts we know what matters. We cannot hope only to leave our children a bigger car, a bigger bank account. We must hope to give them a sense of what it means to be a loyal friend, a loving parent, a citizen who leaves his home, his neighborhood and town better than he found it. What do we want the men and women who work with us to say when we are no longer there? That we were more driven to succeed than anyone around us? Or that we stopped to ask if a sick child had gotten better, and stayed a moment there to trade a word of friendship?

No President, no government, can teach us to remember what is best in what we are. But if the man you have chosen to lead this government can make a difference; if he can celebrate the quieter, deeper successes that are made not of gold and silk, but of better hearts and finer souls; if he can do these things, then he must."

President George H. W. Bush
Inaugural Address
January 20, 1989

— 12 —

THE ELECTION OF 1992

*Population of the United States: **255.46 million***
*Number of eligible voters: **189.04 million***
*Percent of those eligible who voted: **55.2***
*Percent of television saturation in U.S. households: **98***

SETTING THE STAGE

As usual in a presidential election year, economic indicators were used to predict how the incumbent would fare in a re-election bid. On January 29, 1992, President Bush's proposed budget contained a $352 billion deficit. By October, the unemployment rate was 7.4 percent. And on October 9, the Dow Jones industrial average hit the year's low of 3136.58. The gross domestic product (GDP) had increased 3.9 percent in the third quarter, but measures of consumer confidence mirrored the year's other indicators and remained low. The national debt of the United States was now over $3 trillion. It had been $735 billion at the beginning of 1981.

In early 1991, the U.S. military led an international effort in debilitating the Iraqi military forces and repelling them from Kuwait. The success of the U.S. mission in the Persian Gulf brought President Bush great popularity at home in the aftermath of the war, and it looked as if he would be unbeatable in a re-election bid. In October of that year, although it had gone down some since the end of the Iraqi conflict, Bush's popularity remained high.

Facing a Democratically controlled Congress, Bush vetoed 45 bills; only one, a cable television regulation bill, passed over his veto.

In 1992, violence, burning and looting occurred in Los Angeles after a Simi Valley, California, jury acquitted four police officers accused of beating a black man named Rodney King. Following the civil disturbances, Bush agreed to $1.3 billion in grants and loans for the area's businesses and residences.

On July 3, Bush signed into law a measure extending jobless benefits from 26 weeks to 52 weeks. On March 5, The House Ethics Committee reported that more than 350 current and former House members had written over 20,000 overdrafts on their accounts at the House bank between July 1988 and October 1991. Public criticism of Congress rose and in 1992, the 27th Amendment to the Constitution, first proposed in 1789, was ratified. The amendment requires at least one intervening election for members of the House of Representatives before Congress can vote itself another salary increase.

Also in 1992, a federal jury convicted Charles H. Keating Jr. for his activities as head of the Lincoln Savings and Loan Association and ordered him to pay restitution claims of over $3 billion. Before the year was out, two grand juries indicted former presidential assistant, Clark Clifford, among others for alleged infractions in the Bank of Credit and Commerce International (BCCI) case.

Internationally, President Bush and Russian President Boris Yeltsin declared the end of the Cold War. The Soviet Union disbanded in 1991 and became separate republics. Russia, the largest republic, remained powerful. Bosnia-Herzegovina voted for independence from Yugoslavia on February 29, setting off a civil war in the Balkans. In South Africa, anti-apartheid leader Nelson Mandela and President F. W. de Klerk initiated efforts to end white rule and years of conflict over apartheid. And on July 10, 1992, Panama's former military leader, Manuel Noriega, was sentenced to 40 years in U.S. prisons for his involvement in international drug trading.

THE CANDIDATES AND THE ISSUES

ARKANSAS GOVERNOR WILLIAM JEFFERSON CLINTON, THE DEMOCRATIC PARTY CANDIDATE

Clinton was born on August 19, 1946, in Hope, Arkansas. He married Hillary Rodham on October 11, 1975. They had one daughter, Chelsea.

Bill Clinton graduated from Georgetown University in Washington, D.C., in 1968. He spent two years in England at Oxford University as a Rhodes Scholar. After graduating from the Yale University law school in 1973, he taught at the University of Arkansas law school and began a political career.

Clinton was elected attorney general for the state of Arkansas, serving from 1977 to 1979. In 1978, at the age of 32, he was elected governor of Arkansas and held that office from 1979 to 1981. He was defeated in his 1980 bid for re-election. Clinton came back to win the gubernatorial race in 1982. He was re-elected in 1984, 1986, 1988 and 1990, serving until 1993.

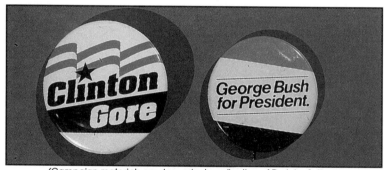

(Campaign materials courtesy private collection of Dr. John Sullivan, University of Virginia/Photo by Paul Kennedy.)

PRESIDENT GEORGE BUSH, THE REPUBLICAN PARTY CANDIDATE

(Bush's biography is in chapter eleven.)

HENRY ROSS PEROT, INDEPENDENT CANDIDATE

Perot was born in Texarkana, Texas, on June 27, 1930. He attended a junior college in Texarkana and graduated from the U.S. Naval Academy in 1953. He served in the Navy from 1953 to 1957.

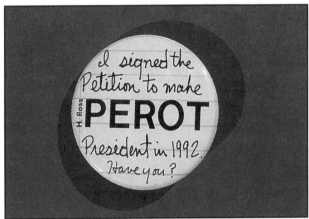

(Campaign materials courtesy private collection of Dr. John Sullivan,
University of Virginia/Photo by Paul Kennedy.)

Perot was a salesman with IBM. From 1957 to 1984, he developed Electronic Data Systems into a company worth $2.5 billion. In 1984 the company was bought by General Motors, and Perot stayed with the merged operation until 1986. Perot remained in private business and did not run for political office until 1992.

After the 1992 election, Perot continued to manage his business interests and coordinated the establishment of "United We Stand America" organizations in all 50 states.

THE ISSUES

Candidates had to address a wide range of issues that concerned voters in 1992: the economy, jobs, government deficits, health care, crime, family values, taxes, abortion, education, international relations, energy resources and the environment. The economy, however, became the central issue of the campaign.

If elected, President Bush planned to continue his policies. His campaign underscored the need for a Republican Congress to work with him. Bush emphasized family values and his opposition to abortion. Vice President Dan Quayle said that the breakdown in family values caused America's societal problems. In a speech on May 19, he pointed to popular television show "Murphy Brown" as an example of social decline, and cited the program's central character, an unwed mother, for "mocking the importance of fathers."

The speech spurred a lot of public response and media attention on both sides of the issue.

Arkansas Governor Bill Clinton promised a new approach to traditional Democratic programs such as welfare and national health care. And H. Ross Perot mounted the strongest independent or third-party candidacy since Theodore Roosevelt in 1912. Perot campaigned for the return of government to the people.

Bill Clinton, Democrat

Clinton opposed four more years of "trickle-down economics" and advocated "invest and growth" policies instead of "tax and spend" programs. He wanted to create good jobs at fair wages. He favored middle-class tax relief and a tax increase for those earning over $200,000. He urged reform of the welfare system to move people out of their dependence on the government and into the work force. Clinton wanted to create a national health insurance program that would provide basic health care to all Americans. He opposed the legalization of drugs, and he supported "choice" in the abortion issue.

The Democratic candidate advocated a strong mobile defense. He said the United States should consider lifting the arms embargo on Bosnia. Clinton supported a cut in defense spending consistent with diminishing Cold War threats and conversion of the savings into technology.

George Bush, Republican

The president's "Agenda for American Renewal" advocated training for displaced workers and increased business investment. He opposed "Mondale-type...tax and spend" policies and Perot's gasoline tax proposal. Bush favored a reduction in the capital gains tax and vowed to veto any tax increases. He favored a constitutional amendment banning abortion and opposed the legalization of drugs.

Bush spoke out against committing American troops anywhere in the world without a clear mission and a plan for bringing them home. He opposed any return to isolationism in international matters and opposed proposals to isolate China. President Bush favored efforts to negotiate nuclear disarmament agreements.

H. Ross Perot, independent

Perot campaigned on two main themes: deficit reduction and returning government to the American people. The businessman called on Americans to face the "harsh reality" of their economic prospects and to share "the sacrifice" necessary to balance the budget and rebuild America's economic power. He suggested raising the gasoline tax 50 cents over five years. He supported building the economic infrastructure of the country and removing needless regulations imposed on small-business operators. Perot wanted to make the American "melting pot" of ethnic diversity a strength and not a weakness. He favored the conversion of American industries into the "industries of tomorrow," but was opposed to international trade agreements like NAFTA. He was against legalizing drugs.

The Campaign

By the end of 1990, no Democrat had formally announced a challenge to the Republican president. Bush's popularity ratings were so high after the conflict in the Persian Gulf that prudence dictated a wait-and-see strategy. However, as the summer of 1991 wore on and the economy sputtered, the president's political armor began to look penetrable.

Entering the 1992 election year, the president still appeared to be at the top of his game. The two Democrats most likely to have the national recognition and resources to take on a popular incumbent, New York Governor Mario Cuomo and New Jersey Senator Bill Bradley, both declined to run.

On February 12, when President Bush formally announced that he would seek re-election, he knew he faced a challenge within his own party from Patrick Buchanan, syndicated columnist, conservative television commentator and former Nixon White House aide. In New Hampshire's primary on February 18, the president held off Buchanan's effort, winning 53 percent to 37 percent of the vote. He then defeated Buchanan by a two-to-one margin in Georgia on March 3. On "Super Tuesday," Bush won all of the contests in which he and Buchanan were both on the ballot. Buchanan exceeded 30 percent of the vote only in Florida and Rhode Island. Support for Buchanan to challenge his own party's incumbent was driven by the perception of a poor economy. Those issues were to play a part in the general election as well.

The Democrats had several potential candidates. Jerry Brown, former governor of California and a candidate in the previous presidential primaries, announced early and employed, perhaps, the most innovative campaign tactic. Brown used an "800" telephone number to solicit contributions of $100 or less from "ordinary" citizens. With the calls he received, he could also determine voter interests, enlist volunteers and develop valuable, targeted mailing lists.

He and the other candidates in this election used other new forums in the campaign—satellites, televised "town meetings" between the candidates and "the people," talk show appearances and the Internet—all emphasizing increased audience participation.

Other candidates in the Democratic primaries were Arkansas Governor Bill Clinton, former Massachusetts Senator Paul Tsongas, Nebraska Senator Robert Kerrey and Iowa Senator Tom Harkin. Virginia Governor Douglas Wilder briefly contemplated entering the contest, but decided against it.

Clinton ran as a "new" Democrat who wanted to reduce federal intervention into state governance. Tsongas wanted more fiscal responsibility on the part of the government and offered an economic program intended to get the deficit under control. Brown argued for policies that would reduce the influence of the wealthy elite on government. Harkin embraced traditional Democratic New Deal politics. And Senator Kerrey, a Vietnam veteran, offered political and military experience.

As expected, Iowa Senator Tom Harkin won his home state's caucuses on February 10. In the New Hampshire primary, former Senator Tsongas of neighboring Massachusetts won with 33 percent of the vote, topping Clinton, who came in second with 25 percent. Governor Clinton called his finish a victory and labeled himself "the comeback kid." The name fit Clinton's youthful, energetic image and some in the media picked up on this theme. Clinton won Georgia on March 3, and on Super Tuesday, March 10, he swept the Southern primaries. Tsongas took two more New England states, his home state of Massachusetts and Rhode Island. On June 2, Clinton won six primaries including the largest delegate prize, California.

At the height of the primary season, Texan Ross Perot unexpectedly announced on CNN's "Larry King Live" that he would accept the will of the American people: If they wanted him to run and if they put him on the ballot in all 50 states, he would run. Perot was the first independent candidate ever to be in the lead against the traditional major-party candidates in public-opinion polls.

Bush and Clinton, by the time of the convention, had run in 32 primaries, and Perot was yet to be tested by the ballot. His quick rise was attributed to his posture as an agent for change. The public response to Perot told the other campaigns that "change" worked, and the word began appearing frequently in all the candidates' literature and advertising. Once again it was an asset to be running from the "outside" against Washington. Many Americans agreed with Perot's criticism of a governmental structure that had created a near $4 trillion federal debt, and many embraced his bite-the-bullet proposals.

THE DEMOCRATIC NATIONAL CONVENTION, NEW YORK, NEW YORK, JULY 13 TO JULY 16

At their 41st national convention, held at Madison Square Garden, the Democrats nominated Arkansas Governor Bill Clinton and Senator Albert Gore Jr. from Tennessee as their presidential and vice-presidential candidates. In choosing Gore, the party did not try to balance Clinton's Southern base with someone from a different region. It was the first time in recent presidential elections that a major party had selected two candidates who represented the South.

Coming out of the Democratic convention, Clinton received a noticeable popularity bump from two events: the Democrats' successful presentation of party unity and the temporary withdrawal of independent candidate Ross Perot. For the first time in the contest, Clinton led both Bush and Perot in the polls. Recalling the costly failure of Dukakis to follow up on his postconvention lead in 1988, Clinton, Gore and their families kept the momentum by almost immediately launching an eight-state bus tour through the country's heartland.

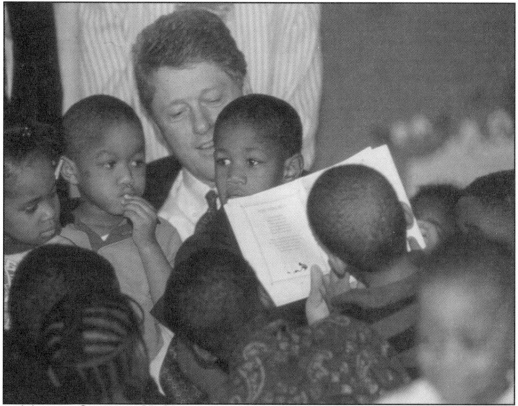

Arkansas Governor Bill Clinton ran in the 1992 election as a "New Democrat,"
favoring middle-class tax relief and reforms of the health and welfare systems.
(Credit: Consolidated News Pictures/Photo by Ron Sachs.)

THE REPUBLICAN NATIONAL CONVENTION, HOUSTON, TEXAS, AUGUST 17 TO AUGUST 20

Just before the convention, a Gallup Poll showed that 37 percent of Republicans believed Bush should replace Vice President Quayle with another candidate. In the end, the party stayed with the team that had won for them in 1988.

After Pat Buchanan agreed to endorse Bush's re-election, he was given time to address the convention. His speech, and the remarks of some of the other speakers, pointed to abortion, sexual deviancy and the absence of school prayer as evidence of the nation's moral decline.

On July 16, asserting that the Democratic Party had "revitalized itself" at its convention, Perot stopped campaigning. All of a sudden it was a Bush-Clinton contest. Both parties went after the Perot supporters, offering them ideas similar to Perot's. In an attempt to boost Bush's bid for re-election, Secretary of State James A. Baker III resigned on August 23 to direct the president's campaign.

By September 8, Perot's supporters had his name certified on all 50 ballots. At the beginning of October, he was back in the race, campaigning on reducing the deficit and minimizing the influence of special interests. Perot said that the American debt was growing at a rate of about $1 billion every day and offered a pamphlet called "United We Stand," instructing Americans "How We Can Take Back Our Country." He continued as a viable and visible candidate and was included in the presidential debates held in October.

National recognition of Ross Perot was enhanced by his high showing in public opinion polls, his television "infomercials" and the fact that his supporters worked zealously in every state to put him on the ballot. Perot chose Admiral James Bond Stockdale to be his running mate. Stockdale had been a prisoner of war in Vietnam and received a congressional medal of honor.

"It's the economy, stupid," a sign prominently displayed in Clinton's political headquarters in Little Rock, Arkansas, reminded Clinton and his campaign staff to focus on the election's biggest issue. A commercial and a biography, both called "The Man from Hope," referred to the candidate's small hometown and extolled his achievements. Clinton's running mate, Al Gore, and Gore's young family, served to accentuate the call for "New Leadership" and the need for change. James Carville and other Clinton advisors urged Clinton to campaign vigorously, and he did. Events like his bus trip were intended to illustrate the vigor of baby boomers as candidates and provided abundant opportunities for interviews in small towns throughout America. The first trip began in New York after the convention and lasted six days, continuing through New Jersey, Pennsylvania, West Virginia, Kentucky, Indiana, Ohio, Illinois and

Missouri. The second trip lasted three days, beginning in St. Louis and continuing to Minneapolis along the Mississippi River.

The Bush campaign had trouble staying with its message, in part because Bush's success had been in international affairs but the American people wanted to hear about his domestic plans. Bush argued, as other incumbents had before him, that he had contributed to the general peace in the world and also that the threat of nuclear war had been reduced. He cited the end of the Cold War, the breakdown of Communist control in Eastern Europe and better relations with Russia. He blamed his domestic woes on a Congress controlled by the Democrats.

TELEVISION AND THE CAMPAIGN

By 1992, new technologies had changed the election process. Candidates now sent their messages directly to the voters, bypassing party leaders and the influence of the national parties. The marriage of computers and television brought computer-generated interactive television to the campaigns. Cable television and computerized mailings provided tools to target specific voters and demographic groups. Campaigns produced and provided video cassettes to potential supporters. The Clinton campaign used this costly tactic in the important New Hampshire primary. "Fax broadcasts" were also a way candidates sent their message simultaneously to a large pool of media and voters. In addition, Clinton's more broadly televised commercials gave a telephone number where people could request a campaign book outlining "Bill Clinton's Plan For Change." Clinton was also one of the first to use the Internet as a campaign device, illustrating the young candidate's interest in new technologies. Through on-line services and electronic mail, the candidates were able to disseminate information and speak to computer users all over the country.

It also seemed to be the year of the televised "call-in show," in which candidates could engage the public in direct conversation. The widespread use of satellites allowed campaigns to transmit to specific cities from a central location; thus the tarmac campaign, the brief replacement of the whistle-stop canvass, moved into the television studio.

Due to the increased importance of fundraising and the early primaries, candidates in recent election cycles have generally announced earlier than in past elections. Perot, however, spent his own money. From early October, Perot spent over a million dollars each day, much of it going for television time on the various networks. A series of 30-minute "infomercials" featuring Perot and his charts-and-graphs instruction on the economic dilemma faced by the United States in approaching the 21st century drew in large numbers of viewers. Since he was not using public funds, billionaire Ross Perot was not subject to the spending limits faced by the party candidates. Nor did he have to devote his time to fundraising efforts. Perot had other advantages: He had no competition for the nomination; he received free publicity from media talk shows and he was the first independent candidate to be invited to share the debate dais with both major-party candidates.

Thought to be trailing behind Clinton, George Bush agreed to debate, and the three candidates—Clinton, Bush and Perot—met for three 90-minute debates. In the first debate, at Washington University in St. Louis, Missouri, on October 11, Clinton held his own. The second debate, in Richmond, Virginia, on October 15, seemed to go in Clinton's favor. Reaction shots of President Bush as he looked at his watch during the telecast suggested detachment. Clinton, on the other hand, created a sense of intimacy by using the U-shape seating arrangement to his advantage and walking into the audience. In the final debate, at Michigan State University in East Lansing, on October 19, all the candidates basically held to their previously stated positions. In general, the presidential debates in 1992 did not change votes, but they did buttress Clinton's small lead.

In 1992, C-SPAN's cameras again covered the candidates from announcements through caucuses, primaries, conventions and on to Election Day. They followed candidates to factory entrances and county fairs, onto production lines and fishing piers and into seafood processing plants, construction pits, diners and school classrooms. The network held extended open-phone sessions so viewers could express their views or talk with the candidates and campaign staff. Additionally, C-SPAN provided time for more than 30 other announced presidential candidates, thus including those who could not get on the same dais with Bush, Clinton and Perot.

ABC, CBS, NBC and PBS continued covering all aspects of the campaign during their nightly newscasts and election specials. The more extensive coverage by CNN and C-SPAN, including C-SPAN's gavel-to-gavel coverage of the conventions, allowed the other networks to vary and target their coverage. Other networks, like MTV and its "Rock the Vote" effort, provided election programming that generated interest. Voter turnout was up over 5 percent from the previous election.

◆ ◆ ◆

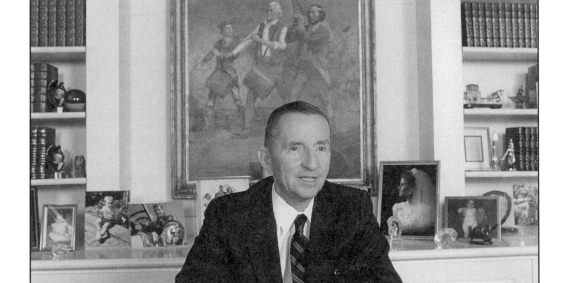

Billionaire businessman Ross Perot entered the 1992 presidential race as an independent, spending over a million dollars of his own money on the campaign each day. (Courtesy United We Stand America.)

THE RESULTS

In an election with the largest voter turnout in recent years, Bill Clinton defeated President George Bush, winning 43 percent to Bush's 37 percent of the popular vote. Only William Howard Taft's 1912 total of 23 percent of the popular vote was lower for an incumbent president. Clinton won states in all sections of the country. He swept the West Coast states, the Northeast and strands of the Midwest. Bush won some of the Midwestern states and did well in the Southeast. Clinton won 370 electoral votes to Bush's 168 votes. Clinton edged Bush among women voters, received a large majority of black votes and gained a significant majority of those identified as "single parents."

With the election of Bill Clinton, one party held the partisan advantage in both the White House and Congress for the first time since 1980. The Democrats maintained a 56 seat to 44 seat advantage in the Senate. In the House of Representatives, Republicans gained nine seats, but remained the minority party with 176 seats to 258 seats for the Democrats.

The Perot candidacy may have opened an opportunity for Clinton in Colorado, Montana, Nevada and New Mexico. Clinton was the first Democratic presidential candidate to win those states since Lyndon Johnson in 1964. Perot gained about 19 percent of the popular vote, an impressive showing for a first-time independent candidate, and gathered a group of committed supporters who stayed with him. After the election, he coordinated "United We Stand America" political groups around the country to influence the choice of future candidates and issues.

1992

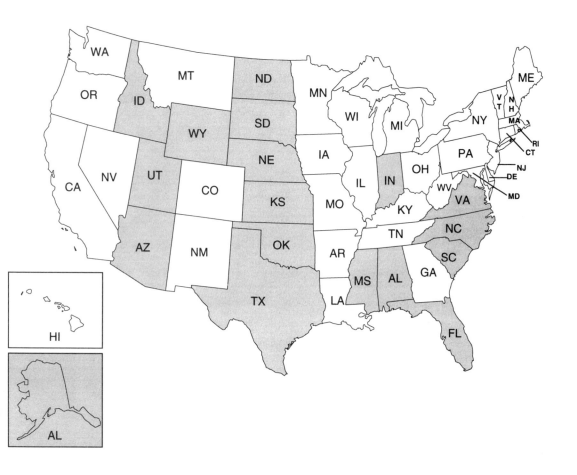

Clinton (Democrat)
Bush (Republican)

POSTSCRIPT

In the election of 1994 the Republicans regained control of both houses of Congress for the first time in 40 years. As this book went to press, presidential and congressional campaigns for the 1996 election were already underway and up to 10 Republican candidates were usually invited to early political events. This group included former Secretary of Education Lamar Alexander, media commentator Pat Buchanan, Senate Majority Leader Robert Dole from Kansas, Representative Robert Dornan from California, businessman Malcolm "Steve" Forbes Jr., Senator Phil Gramm from Texas, former Ambassador Alan Keyes, Senator Richard Lugar from Indiana, Senator Arlen Specter from Philadelphia and a businessman named Morry Taylor. California Governor Pete Wilson was a late and short-lived entrant. He had difficulty raising money and left the race after approximately five weeks. Ross Perot announced the creation of a new political party, the Independence Party. Retired General Colin Powell was in the midst of a book tour for his autobiography *My American Journey.* His popularity had many urging him to enter the presidential campaign as either a Republican or independent candidate. While the Republican field was quite crowded, President Clinton appeared to be the only Democratic candidate. By August 1995, the Federal Election Commission had received "Statements of Candidacy" from 166 individuals intending to run for the presidency in 1996.

"Thomas Jefferson believed that to perceive the very foundations of our nation we would need dramatic change from time to time. Well, my fellow Americans, this is our time. Let us embrace it.

Our democracy must be not only the envy of the world but the engine of our own renewal. There is nothing wrong with America that cannot be cured by what is right with America. And so today we pledge an end to the era of deadlock and drift, and a new season of American renewal has begun.

To renew America we must be bold. We must do what no generation has had to do before. We must invest more in our own people—in their jobs and in their future—and at the same time cut our massive debt. And we must do so in a world in which we must compete for every opportunity. It will not be easy. It will require sacrifice. But it can be done and done fairly. Not choosing sacrifice for its own sake, but for our own sake. We must provide for our nation the way a family provides for its children."

President William J. Clinton
Inaugural Address
January 20, 1993

=== 13 ===
OBSERVING THE RULES OF THE ROAD

The road to the White House has advanced far beyond the dirt path of the 1800's or even the two-lane highway of 1948. Now, it is a superhighway, fast-moving and filled with technology and interchanges which may not yet be on the map. This chapter brings into focus some of the changes discussed in this book, so that interested observers can follow the road in this and future elections.

The U.S. electorate continues to grow and change: Alaska and Hawaii were admitted to the union, adding six electoral votes to the 1960 election; citizens of the District of Columbia won the right to vote in national elections with the ratification of the 23rd amendment in 1961; and the 26th amendment, ratified in 1971, lowered the national voting age to 18. In the last generation, the U.S. population has not only grown, it has grown older; rustbelt states lost citizens to the South and southwest; and the percentage of non-white citizens continued to rise. Each of these events and trends have affected the electoral map.

Since the dawn of television, advances in technology and their adaptation to political campaigns seem to occur at dizzying speed. In nearly every election cycle, the growth of technology allows campaigns to find new ways to reach mass audiences and to target specific voting blocs. The first spot advertisements in 1952 have progressed to the paid "infomercials" of 1992. Televised candidate debates emerged in 1960; and in 1992, technology brought private citizens into the debates with the increased use of the town meeting format. The three networks of the 1960 campaign have seen their dominance fractured by the emergence of dozens of satellite-delivered cable networks.

The so-called new technologies will continue to affect presidential politics. Toll-free telephone numbers, rapid reaction polling, low-cost satellite time, and the rise of computer households have already made their marks on recent presidential elections. The 1996 campaign marks the further introduction of the Internet to politics: Candidates, political parties, and grass-roots organizations have established "home pages" on the Internet's World Wide Web.

Despite many changes, there are some constants to watch on the road to the White House: money, the framing of issues, the political parties, use of paid media, news coverage, the importance of key campaign events such as the early primaries, the conventions and the debates, and the quest for 270 electoral votes. What follows is a series of suggestions designed to help you analyze the presidential election process.

THE PRIMARY SEASON

The delegate selection process is now "front-loaded." Of course, there are Iowa and New Hampshire—the first-in-the-nation caucus and primary. However, in 1996, enough other states have moved their primary elections so that by April sufficient delegates could be selected to secure the nomination. Even if you don't live in Iowa or New Hampshire, it is possible to track certain aspects of the campaign's early months.

MONEY

In the age of televised campaigning, television time is one of the largest campaign expenditures and candidates need a lot of it to campaign in the early primary states. In the 1996 race, California Governor Pete Wilson, a Republican, was an early casualty because he failed to raise enough money to be competitive in Iowa and New Hampshire. Which candidate raises the most money is also an early indicator of support. Donors are a good guide to a candidate's constituencies. Candidate finance reports are released by the Federal Election Commission on a regular basis. You can usually follow the money in presidential campaigns by carefully reading, listening, and watching for the media stories which result from these reports.

CANDIDATES

Since opponents in the early months are party rivals, watch the candidates from the party out of power for "ad hominem" attacks— criticism of the person rather than their policies. It is likely that some of the charges leveled at the successful nominee during the primary season will resurface during the general campaign as criticism from the opposing party.

ADVISORS

Many times the media will report who the campaigns have signed on as consultants and which campaigns they organized in the past. In the compressed time frame of primary season, campaign advisors can be critical. Recall the role Clinton advisor James Carville played in 1992's New Hampshire primary, responding to shape the story when Mr. Clinton's military service issue broke, as well as Bush advisor James Baker's efforts to boost Bush's campaign in the general election.

NEW TECHNOLOGIES

Look for the introduction of new technologies. In 1992, Democratic contender Jerry Brown introduced the toll-free number during the primary season. By the general campaign, it had been freely adopted by the campaigns of Ross Perot, Bill Clinton, and George Bush.

THE CONVENTIONS

Because of the delegate selection process, brokered conventions seem relegated to the past. There are, however, a few things to observe in this stage of the process. The vice-presidential selection will be made public; party platforms are decided and released, and the conventions are the first formal introductions many Americans have to the party nominees.

SITE SELECTION

Note, first of all, the cities selected to hold the conventions. Conventions bring money and visibility to a state and parties usually make choices that appeal to key constituencies and/or help secure Electoral College votes.

CONVENTION SCHEDULE

The schedule is another key to party and candidate constituencies. Even the musical selections are chosen in an effort to appeal to certain voting blocs. Watch who is selected to speak—and when: prime-time exposure is carefully managed by current-day campaigns. The people chosen to deliver keynote speeches, to enter names into nomination, to act as surrogates for the nominees at press conferences are all keys to how the campaign hopes to position itself for the general campaign.

ACCEPTANCE SPEECH

The acceptance speech is designed to set the thematic direction of the campaign. Look for the post-speech analysis and watch as the candidates return to the issues during the fall campaign.

THE GENERAL CAMPAIGN

Nominees now generally "hit the road" right out of the convention. Every day is important in the search for 270 Electoral College votes. Watch which states a candidate visits regularly; you will soon discern their Electoral College strategy. Paid and free media become critical to the outcome. And the candidate debates often become defining moments of the campaign.

THIRD PARTY CANDIDATES

Their viability now becomes critical to the outcome. The ways in which the candidates of the major parties respond to independent or third-party candidates can be telling. The party most likely to benefit from the presence of a viable third-party candidate will often work hardest to foster their participation in the process.

MESSAGE OF THE DAY

The "message of the day" has become an accepted campaign strategy. Look for campaign events as they are covered in long-form on the new media—C-SPAN and CNN—and in the broadcast networks' nightly newscasts. Can you spot the campaigns' attempts to control the message?

DEBATES

The debates are another forum in which the candidates attempt to control the message. Listen carefully to the answers delivered by the candidates—do they match the question or does the candidate attempt to move the message back to a central theme of his campaign? Watch for the "defining moment" of the debate—each candidate hopes to have a positive one. Listen to the "spin doctors" who work the media after the debates to see how the advisors hope to position their candidate's performance.

PAID MEDIA

Paid media increases in frequency as Election Day draws near. Look for the candidates' positions and how they change over the course of the campaign. Are advertisements "positive"—supporting the qualities of the nominee, or "negative"—attacking the opponent personally or politically? Themes should be apparent consistent with the themes laid out by the candidate during the convention. Watch for support ads sponsored by the parties and special interest groups. They will be a key to issues and constituencies important to the candidates in the future.

SIGNIFICANT EVENTS

Most campaigns will have one or several significant events which alter the course of the election. It is hard to predict whether this will come during the convention, the debates or during an event—or set of events—during the general election.

NEW TECHNOLOGIES

Look for new technologies, especially those pioneered during the primary season to make their mark in the campaigns. In 1992, the "town hall" carried by satellite, the candidate call-in program, and the paid "infomercial" all became hallmarks of the general campaign.

The Road to the White House Since Television's historical look at elements, old and new, in the campaigns since 1948 provides a framework for looking at future elections. Television, barely a factor in 1948, is a fixture of the modern campaign. Candidates in the 1996 election and beyond will undoubtedly draw upon the successful techniques of prior campaigns. Yet the emergence of new technologies and new applications of older technologies and the vagaries of each election cycle continue to influence the results. As much as an individual candidate hopes to control the campaign, the volatility of the race for the presidency persists. That is why American presidential politics continues to be a subject of worldwide interest.

APPENDIX

The Electoral College

The Constitution of the United States mandates that the president be chosen by the electors within the Electoral College. Each state nominates their own electors, one for each senator and representative representing that state in Congress. The District of Columbia gets three electors despite having no voting members of Congress. Each political party chooses a slate of electors pledged to that party's presidential and vice-presidential candidates.

The names of the electors usually do not appear on the ballots. On the first Monday after the second Wednesday in December, after the popular votes have been received on Election Day, the electors gather in their state capitals to cast their ballots. The slate of electors whose candidate wins more popular votes in a given state than any other candidate is authorized to cast all the electoral votes of that state in the Electoral College.

The votes are then certified by the respective states and sent to Congress. There, on January 6, the president of the Senate opens the certificates and has them counted in the presence of both houses of Congress to confirm the results. This is usually just a formality as the electoral votes should reflect the popular votes. The electors are not pledged to vote with the popular vote and the party, but they invariably do.

In the event that no candidate receives a majority of the electoral votes, the House of Representatives is authorized to choose a president from among the three leading candidates. The representatives from each state vote in a bloc, not as individuals. A majority is needed. A vice president may be chosen in the Senate from the two vice-presidential candidates with the most votes, by the senators voting as individuals.

Electoral Votes Per State For 1996 Election

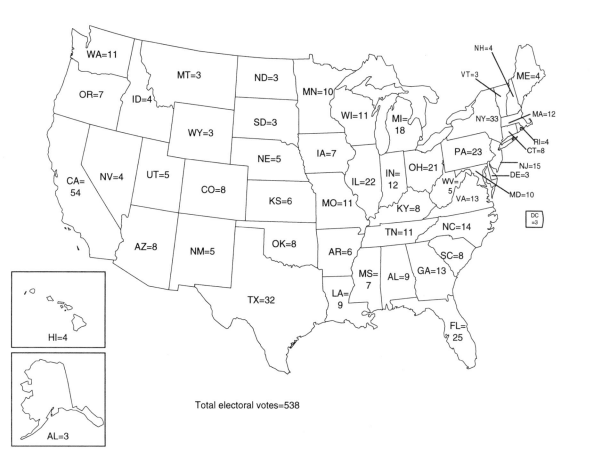

WA=11
MT=3
ND=3
MN=10
NH=4
VT=3
ME=4
OR=7
ID=4
WI=11
NY=33
MA=12
SD=3
MI=18
RI=4
CT=8
WY=3
NE=5
IA=7
PA=23
NJ=15
CA=54
NV=4
UT=5
IL=22
IN=12
OH=21
DE=3
CO=8
KS=6
MO=11
WV=5
VA=13
MD=10
KY=8
DC=3
AZ=8
NM=5
OK=8
TN=11
NC=14
AR=6
SC=8
MS=7
AL=9
GA=13
TX=32
LA=9
FL=25

HI=4

AL=3

Total electoral votes=538

Distribution of Electoral Votes 1948-1996

State	1948	1952*1956*1960	1964*1968	1972*1976*1980	1984*1988	1992*1996
Alabama	11	11	10	9	9	9
Alaska	n/a	3	3	3	3	3
Arizona	4	4	5	6	7	8
Arkansas	9	8	6	6	6	6
California	25	32	40	45	47	54
Colorado	6	6	6	7	8	8
Connecticut	8	8	8	8	8	8
Delaware	3	3	3	3	3	3
District of Columbia	n/a	n/a	3	3	3	3
Florida	8	10	14	17	21	25
Georgia	12	12	12	12	12	13
Hawaii	n/a	3	4	4	4	4
Idaho	4	4	4	4	4	4
Illinois	28	27	26	26	24	22
Indiana	13	13	13	13	12	12
Iowa	10	10	9	8	8	7
Kansas	8	8	7	7	7	6
Kentucky	11	10	9	9	9	8
Louisiana	10	10	10	10	10	9
Maine	5	5	4	4	4	4
Maryland	8	9	10	10	10	10
Massachusetts	16	16	14	14	13	12
Michigan	19	20	21	21	20	18
Minnesota	11	11	10	10	10	10
Mississippi	9	8	7	7	7	7
Missouri	15	13	12	12	11	11
Montana	4	4	4	4	4	3
Nebraska	6	6	5	5	5	5
Nevada	3	3	3	3	4	4
New Hampshire	4	4	4	4	4	4
New Jersey	16	16	17	17	16	15
New Mexico	4	4	4	4	5	5
New York	47	45	43	41	36	33
North Carolina	14	14	13	13	13	14
North Dakota	4	4	4	3	3	3
Ohio	25	25	26	25	23	21
Oklahoma	10	8	8	8	8	8
Oregon	6	6	6	6	7	7
Pennsylvania	35	32	29	27	25	23
Rhode Island	4	4	4	4	4	4
South Carolina	8	8	8	8	8	8
South Dakota	4	4	4	4	3	3
Tennessee	12	11	11	10	11	11
Texas	23	24	25	26	29	32
Utah	4	4	4	4	5	5
Vermont	3	3	3	3	3	3
Virginia	11	12	12	12	12	13
Washington	8	9	9	9	10	11
West Virginia	8	8	7	6	6	5
Wisconsin	12	12	12	11	11	11
Wyoming	3	3	3	3	3	3

Note: Alaska and Hawaii figures apply since the election of 1960 only.

Source: Congressional Quarterly, *Presidential Elections 1789-1992.*
Washington, D.C.: Congressional Quarterly Inc., 1995.

General Election Results 1948-1992

Election Year	Candidates	Popular Votes	Percent of Popular Vote	Electoral Votes	Number of States
1948	Harry S. Truman (D)	24,179,345	49.60	303	28
	Thomas E. Dewey (R)	21,991,291	45.10	189	16
	Strom Thurmond (SR)	1,176,125	2.40	39	4
	Henry Wallace (P)	1,157,326	2.40	0	0
1952	Dwight D. Eisenhower (R)	33,936,234	55.10	442	39
	Adlai Stevenson (D)	27,314,992	44.40	89	9
1956	Dwight D. Eisenhower (R)	35,590,472	57.00	457	41
	Adlai Stevenson (D)	26,022,752	42.00	73	7
1960	John F. Kennedy (D)	34,226,731	49.70	303	22
	Richard M. Nixon (R)	34,108,157	49.50	219	26
1964	Lyndon B. Johnson (D)	43,129,566	61.10	486	45
	Barry Goldwater (R)	27,178,188	38.50	52	6
1968	Richard M. Nixon (R)	31,785,480	43.40	301	32
	Hubert Humphrey (D)	31,275,166	42.70	191	14
	George Wallace (AI)	9,906,473	13.50	46	5
1972	Richard M. Nixon (R)	47,169,911	60.07	520	49
	George McGovern (D)	27,170,383	37.50	17	2
	John Schmitz (A)	1,099,482	1.40	0	0
1976	Jimmy Carter (D)	40,830,763	50.10	297	24
	Gerald Ford (R)	39,147,793	48.00	240	27
1980	Ronald Reagan (R)	43,904,153	50.70	489	44
	Jimmy Carter (D)	35,483,883	41.00	49	7
	John Anderson (I)	5,720,060	6.60	0	0
1984	Ronald Reagan (R)	54,455,075	58.80	525	49
	Walter Mondale (D)	37,577,185	40.60	13	2
1988	George Bush (R)	48,886,097	53.40	426	40
	Michael Dukakis (D)	41,809,074	45.60	111	11
1992	Bill Clinton (D)	44,909,326	43.00	370	33
	George Bush (R)	39,103,882	37.40	168	18
	H. Ross Perot (I)	19,741,657	18.90	0	0

Note: (D) Democrat; (R) Republican; (I) Independent; (SR) States' Rights; (P) Progressive; (AI) American Independent; (A) American.

Number of states includes the District of Columbia 1964-1992. In the election of 1960, Harry S. Byrd (D) won most of the electoral votes in Alabama and Mississippi, but did not reach the one-million popular vote figure. The total number of states for Kennedy and Nixon, 48, reflects Byrd's exclusion from this table.

Source: Congressional Quarterly, *Presidential Elections 1789-1992*.
Washington, D.C.: Congressional Quarterly Inc., 1995.

Congressional Election Results 1946-1994

Election Year	Congress Elected	House Members Elected Dem.	Rep.	Misc.	House Gains/Losses Dem.	Rep.	Senate Party Lineup Dem.	Rep.	Misc.	Senate Gains/Losses Dem.	Rep.
1946	80th	188	246	1	-53	+55	45	51	0	-11	+11
1948	81st	263	171	1	+76	-76	54	42	0	+9	-9
1950	82nd	235	199	1	-27	+27	49	47	0	-5	+5
1952	83rd	213	221	1	-24	+24	47	48	1	-2	+2
1954	84th	232	203	0	+19	-18	48	47	1	+2	-2
1956	85th	234	201	0	+2	-2	49	47	0	0	0
1958	86th	283	153	0	+49	-48	64	34	0	+15	-13
1960	87th	263	174	0	-20	+21	64	36	0	-2	+2
1962	88th	258	176	1	-4	0	68	32	0	+4	-4
1964	89th	295	140	0	+38	-37	68	32	0	+2	-2
1966	90th	248	187	0	-48	+48	64	36	0	-3	+3
1968	91st	243	192	0	-7	+7	58	42	0	-5	+5
1970	92nd	255	180	0	+12	-12	55	45	0	-2	+2
1972	93rd	244	191	0	-13	+13	57	43	0	+2	-2
1974	94th	291	144	0	+48	-48	61	38	0	+3	-4
1976	95th	292	143	0	+2	-2	62	38	0	0	0
1978	96th	277	158	0	-12	+12	59	41	0	-3	+3
1980	97th	243	192	0	-33	+33	47	53	0	-12	+12
1982	98th	269	166	0	+26	-26	46	54	0	0	0
1984	99th	253	182	0	-15	+15	47	53	0	+2	-2
1986	100th	258	177	0	+5	-5	55	45	0	+8	-8
1988	101st	260	175	0	+3	-3	55	45	0	+1	-1
1990	102nd	267	167	1	+8	-9	56	44	0	+1	-1
1992	103rd	258	176	1	-9	+9	56	44	0	0	0
1994	104th	203	231	1	-53	+53	47	53	0	-9	+9

Note:
In 1958, Alaska elected two Democrats to the Senate after winning statehood.
In 1962, Democratic Representative Clem Miller of California died. Don Clausen, a Republican, won the vacancy in a special election.
In 1974, the race for the New Hampshire seat, between Democrat John A. Durkin and Republican Louis C. Wyman resulted in a virtual tie. Durkin won a special election in September 1975.

Source: Congressional Quarterly, *The Weekly Report, Special Supplement*. Congressional Quarterly, Inc., February 29, 1992.

Population and Participation in Elections

Election Years	1.Total U.S. Population (in millions)	2.VAP: Voting Age Population (in millions)	3.Actual Voters (in millions)	Percent of VAP
1948	146.63	95.57	48.79	51.10
1950	152.27	98.13	40.34	41.10
1952	157.55	99.93	61.55	61.60
1954	163.03	102.08	42.58	41.70
1956	168.90	104.52	62.03	59.30
1958	174.88	106.45	45.82	43.00
1960	180.67	109.67	68.84	62.80
1962	186.54	112.95	51.27	45.40
1964	191.89	114.09	70.65	61.90
1966	196.56	116.64	52.91	45.40
1968	200.71	120.29	73.21	60.90
1970	205.05	124.49	54.17	43.50
1972	209.90	140.78	77.72	55.20
1974	213.85	146.34	52.50	35.90
1976	218.04	152.31	81.56	53.50
1978	222.59	158.37	55.33	34.90
1980	227.73	164.60	86.52	52.60
1982	232.19	169.94	64.52	38.00
1984	236.35	174.47	92.65	53.10
1986	240.65	178.57	59.62	33.40
1988	245.02	182.78	91.60	50.10
1990	249.91	185.81	61.51	33.10
1992	255.46	189.04	104.43	55.2

Note:
1.1948 figures from *Historical Abstract of the U.S. Colonial Times to 1970*, Annual Population Estimates, U.S. Department of Commerce (This figure is not statistically comparable with 1950-1992). Figures estimated as of July 1.
2.Figures estimated as of November and include: Resident population (including Armed Forces and aliens) 21 years and over, 1948-1970, except as noted, and 18 years old and over thereafter. Alaska and Hawaii excluded prior to 1960. District of Columbia is included in votes cast for president beginning in 1964 and in votes cast for representatives beginning in 1972. Population 18 and over in Georgia, 1948-1970, and in Kentucky, 1956-1970; 19 and over in Alaska and 20 and over in Hawaii, 1960-1970.
3.Source: Years 1948-58 from U.S. Congress, Clerk of the House, *Statistics of the Presidential and Congressional Election*, biennial.
Source (Except as noted above): U.S. Bureau of the Census, Current Population Reports, (Compiled in Statistical Abstract of the United States 1994, *The National Data Book*, U.S. Department of Commerce, Economics and Statistical Administration, Bureau of the Census, 114th ed., Table No. 449, and America Votes, Chevy Chase, Md: Election Research Center, biennial.

Economic Indicators 1947-1994

Years	Unemployment Rate (Percent of civilian labor force)	CPI-U Average All urban consumers (All items) 1982-84=100	Percent Change in CPI-U (Avg.-Avg.)
1947	3.90	22.3	14.4
1948	3.80	24.1	8.10
1949	5.90	23.80	-1.20
1950	5.30	24.10	1.30
1951	3.30	26.00	7.90
1952	3.00	26.50	1.90
1953	2.90	26.70	0.80
1954	5.50	26.90	0.70
1955	4.40	26.80	-0.40
1956	4.10	27.20	1.50
1957	4.30	28.10	3.30
1958	6.80	28.90	2.80
1959	5.50	29.10	0.70
1960	5.50	29.60	1.70
1961	6.70	29.90	1.00
1962	5.50	30.20	1.00
1963	5.70	30.60	1.30
1964	5.20	31.00	1.30
1965	4.50	31.50	1.60
1966	3.80	32.40	2.90
1967	3.80	33.40	3.10
1968	3.60	34.80	4.20
1969	3.50	36.70	5.50
1970	4.90	38.80	5.70
1971	5.90	40.50	4.40
1972	5.80	41.80	3.20
1973	4.90	44.40	6.2
1974	5.60	49.30	11.00
1975	8.50	53.80	9.10
1976	7.7	56.9	5.8
1977	7.1	60.6	6.5
1978	6.10	65.20	7.60
1979	5.80	72.60	11.30
1980	7.10	82.40	13.50
1981	7.60	90.90	10.30
1982	8.70	96.50	6.20
1983	9.60	99.60	3.20
1984	7.50	103.90	4.30
1985	7.20	107.60	3.60
1986	7.00	109.60	1.90
1987	6.20	113.60	3.60
1988	5.50	118.30	4.10
1989	5.30	124.00	4.80
1990	5.50	130.70	5.40
1991	6.70	136.20	4.20
1992	7.40	140.30	3.00
1993	8.80	144.50	3.00
1994	8.10	148.20	2.60

* Note and source on following page.

Note:

Figures for 1953, 1960, 1962, 1972, 1973, 1978 and 1986 are not strictly comparable with prior year data. Data for 1994 is not directly comparable for 1993 and earlier years because of major redesign of Current Population Survey questionnaire and collection methodology and the introduction of 1990 census-based population controls, adjusted for the estimated undercount.

The CPI is a measure of the average change in prices paid by urban consumers for a fixed market basket of goos and services. It is calculated monthly for two population groups, one consisting only of wage earners and clerical workers and the other of all urban families. The all urban families index (CPI-U) is representative of the buying habits of about 80 percent of U.S. population.

Source: U.S. Department of Labor, Bureau of Labor Statistics.

The Growth of Broadcast and Cable Television Households 1948-1992

Presidential Election Years	Total US Households	Total Broadcast Television Households	Percent Broadcast Television Saturation	Total Cable Households	Percent Cable Saturation
1948	39.95	0.172	0.40	-----	-----
1952	44.76	15.30	34.20	0.014	0.30
1956	48.60	34.90	71.80	0.30	0.62
1960	52.50	45.75	87.10	0.65	1.2
1964	55.90	51.60	92.30	1.09	1.90
1968	59.90	56.67	94.60	2.80	4.70
1972	66.28	63.50	95.80	6.00	9.00
1976	73.35	71.47	97.00	10.80	14.70
1980	79.54	78.02	98.00	16.00	20.10
1984	85.43	83.81	98.00	29.00	33.95
1988	90.26	88.55	98.00	44.00	48.75
1992	93.12	91.55	98.00	53.00	56.92

Note:

Percent Cable Saturation compiled using total U.S. households as base.

Source: *Television Factbook*, of Television Digest Reports Annual Factbooks since 1948; Warren Publishing, Washington, D.C. Research product of A.C. Nielson Co./NBC Research Department.

Political Spending 1948-1992

Presidential Election Years	1.Total Political Spending	2.Total Presidential Spending	3.Total Network Political Advertising	4.General Election Broadcasting (Network TV)
1948	-----	-----	-----	-----
1952	140.00	-----	-----	3.00
1956	155.00	-----	-----	6.60
1960	175.00	30.00	-----	10.10
1964	200.00	60.00	-----	17.50
1968	300.00	100.00	-----	27.10
1972	425.00	138.00	24.58	24.60
1976	540.00	160.00	50.84	-----
1980	1200.00	275.00	90.57	-----
1984	1800.00	325.00	153.83	-----
1988	2700.00	500.00	227.90	-----
1992	3220.00	550.00	299.62	-----

Note: All figures in millions.

Source:
1. Alexander, Herbert with Anthony Corrado, *Financing the 1992 Election*, Armonk, N.Y.: M.E. Sharpe, 1995, p. 6.

2. Years 1960-1988 from Alexander, Herbert with Monica Bauer, *Financing the 1988 Election*, Boulder, Colo.: Westview Press, 1991; p. 13 Table 2.2; 1992 figures from Alexander, *Financing the 1992 Election*, p. 5 Table 1.1.

3. Television Bureau of Advertising, New York, 1995.

4. Alexander, Herbert, *Financing the 1972 Election*, Lexington, Mass.: Heath Lexington Books, 1976; p. 324, Table 8.3; 1952 figures from Heard, Alexander, *The Costs of Democracy*, Chapel Hill, N.C.: University of North Carolina Press, 1960, p. 22; 1956-1972 figures from FCC Survey of Political Broadcasting, 1968 Survey, Table 3; 1972 Survey, Table 11.

Viewership and Coverage of Presidential Debates

Election Year	Dates	Times	Locations	Participants	Millions of Viewers
1960	September 26	7:30-8:30 PM (ALL DATES)	Chicago, IL	John F. Kennedy and Richard Nixon	66.4
	October 7		Washington, DC		61.9
	October 13		New York, NY & Hollywood, CA		63.7
	October 21		New York, NY		60.4
1976	September 23	9:30-11:00 PM (ALL DATES)	Philadelphia, PA	Gerald Ford and Jimmy Carter	72.5
	October 6		San Francisco, CA		65.3
	October 22		Williamsburg, VA		59.7
1980	September 21	10:00-11:00 PM	Baltimore, MD	John Anderson and Ronald Reagan and Jimmy Carter* (*Second debate only)	N/A
	October 28	9:30-11:00 PM	Cleveland, OH		71.2
1984	October 7	9:00-10:30 PM (ALL DATES)	Louisville, KY	Ronald Reagan and Walter Mondale	59.1
	October 21		Kansas City, MO		N/A
1988	September 25	8:00 PM	Winston-Salem, NC	George Bush and Michael Dukakis	65
	October 13	9:00 PM	Los Angeles, CA		67
1992	October 11	7:00 PM	St. Louis, MO	Goerge Bush and Bill Clinton and H. Ross Perot	85
	October 15	9:00 PM	Richmond, VA		89
	October 19	7:00 PM	East Lansing, MI		97

Source: Years 1960-1984 from Swerdlow, Joel L. and League of Women Voters, *Presidential Debates 1988 and Beyond*, Washington, D.C.: Congressional Quarterly, Inc., 1987; Years 1988-1992 from Commission on Presidential Debates, Washington, D.C. Viewership figures from A.C. Nielson Research Co.

A NOTE ON SOURCES

*T*he *Road to the White House Since Television* was developed using a variety of primary and secondary sources. Among the primary sources were: videotapes of the conventions since 1948, the available political commercials since 1952, campaign materials from the various elections and the extant campaign videos of the unfolding process. In a book like this one, watching the same television as the voters in a given election season did at the time is a *sine qua non* for the study of elections since the advent of television.

Having grown up in New Hampshire, this author also had an opportunity to witness and participate in the first-in-the-nation presidential primary. This firsthand experience was invaluable in gaining perspective on the process. Further discussions with the people who played a role in the process in New Hampshire and elsewhere have proved instructive and integral to the preparation of this book.

The author has also visited presidential libraries and museums and the depositories for the papers of the defeated candidates, as well as some presidential homes and hometowns. This has helped to round out the study of a given campaign. A museum's or library's choice of what to display and emphasize has proved to be helpful in understanding contemporary views of a candidacy. The following campaign collections have generally been made available to scholars and the public:

Harry S. Truman Library
U.S. Hwy. 24 & Delaware St.
Independence, Mo. 64050-1798
(816) 833-1400

Hubert Humphrey
Minnesota Historical Society
Research Center/Manuscript
Division
345 Kellogg Blvd. West
St. Paul, Minn. 55102-1906
(612) 296-2143

Thomas E. Dewey
University of Rochester
Department of Rare Books and
Special Collections
River Campus
Rochester, N.Y. 14627
(716) 275-4477

George Wallace: Privately Held

George McGovern: Privately
Held

John Schmitz: Privately Held

J. Strom Thurmond
Clemson University/Special
Collections
Clemson, S.C. 29634-3001
(803) 656-3027

Gerald R. Ford Library
1000 Beal Avenue
Ann Arbor, Mich. 48109
(313) 741-2218

Henry Wallace
Iowa State University
Parks Library
Ames, Iowa 50011
(515) 294-4111

Jimmy Carter Library
One Copenhill Avenue
Atlanta, Ga. 30307
(404) 331-3942

Dwight D. Eisenhower Library
Southeast 4th St.
Abilene, Kan. 67410
(913) 263-4751

Ronald Reagan Library
40 Presidential Drive
Simi Valley, Calif. 93065
(805) 522-8444

Adlai E. Stevenson
Princeton University
Seeley G. Mudd Manuscript
Library
Princeton, N.J. 08544
(609) 258-3180

Walter Mondale
Minnesota Historical Society
Research Center-Manuscript
Division
345 Kellogg Blvd. West
St. Paul, Minn. 55102

John F. Kennedy Library
Columbia Point
Boston, Mass. 02125
(617) 929-4500

Bush Presidential Materials
Project
701 University Dr., E. Suite 300
College Station, Texas 77840-1897
(409) 260-9552

Lyndon Baines Johnson Library
and Museum
2313 Red River St.
Austin, Texas 78705
(512) 482-5137

Michael Dukakis
Massachusetts State House
Library
Special Collections
341 State House
Boston, Mass. 02133
(617) 727-2590

Barry Goldwater
Arizona Historical Foundation/
Arizona State University
Hayden Library
Tempe, Ariz. 85287-1006
(602) 965-3283

H. Ross Perot
United We Stand America
P.O. Box 6
Dallas, Texas 75251
(214) 960-9100

Richard Nixon Presidential
Library and Birthplace
18001 Yorba Linda Blvd.
Yorba Linda, Calif. 92686
(714) 993-3393

The Presidential Museum
622 North Lee
Odessa, Texas 79761
(915) 332-7123

The sources that follow are separated by topic to provide readers ready access to books of particular interest. However, the categories are not exclusive and many books could easily be placed in multiple categories.

HISTORY OF ELECTIONS

Boller, Paul F., Jr., *Presidential Campaigns*. New York: Oxford University Press, 1985.

Bush, Gregory, ed., *Campaign Speeches of American Presidential Candidates 1948-1984*. New York: Frederick Ungar Publishing, 1985.

Diamond, Edwin and Stephen Bates, *The Spot: The Rise of Political Advertising on Television*. Third edition. Cambridge, Mass.: The MIT Press, 1992.

Goldinger, Carolyn, ed., *Presidential Elections Since 1789*. Fourth edition. Washington, D.C.: Congressional Quarterly, 1987.

McGuinness, Colleen, ed., *National Party Conventions 1831-1988*. Washington, D.C.: Congressional Quarterly, 1991.

Roseboom, Eugene H. and Alfred H. Eckes, Jr., *A History of Presidential Campaigns: From George Washington to Jimmy Carter*. Fourth edition. New York: Macmillan, 1979.

Shields-West, Eileen, *The World Almanac of Presidential Campaigns*. New York: Pharohs Books, 1992.

White, Theodore H., *America in Search of Itself: The Making of the President 1956-1980*. New York: Harper and Row, 1982.

HISTORY OF MEDIA AND ELECTIONS

Asher, Herbert B., *Presidential Elections and American Politics: Voters, Candidates, and Campaigns Since 1952*. Fifth edition. Pacific Grove, Calif.: Brooks/Cole, 1992.

Joslyn, Richard, *Mass Media and Elections*. Reading, Mass.: Addison-Wesley, 1984.

Melder, Keith, *Hail to the Candidate: Presidential Campaigns From Banners to Broadcasts*. Washington, D.C.: Smithsonian Institution Press, 1992.

Michelson, Sig, *From Whistle Stop to Sound Bite: Four Decades of Politics and Television*. New York: Praeger, 1989.

Reinsch, J. Leonard, *Getting Elected: From Radio and Roosevelt to Television and Reagan*. New York: Hippocrene Books, 1988.

Schlesinger, Arthur Jr., *Running For President: The Candidates and Their Images, 1900-1992*. Volume II. New York: Simon and Schuster, 1994.

Troy, Gil, *See How They Ran: The Changing Role of the Presidential Candidate.* New York: The Free Press, 1991.

HISTORY OF THE MEDIA

Barnouw, Erik, *Tube of Plenty: The Evolution of American Television*. Second revised edition. New York: Oxford University Press, 1990.

Czitrom, Daniel J., *Media and the American Mind: From Morse to McLuhan.* Chapel Hill, N.C.: University of North Carolina Press, 1982.

Jamieson, Kathleen Hall, *Packaging the Presidency: A History and Criticism of Presidential Campaign Advertising*. Second edition. New York: Oxford University Press, 1992.

Kern, Montague, *30-Second Politics: Political Advertising in the Eighties.* New York: Praeger, 1989.

Wattenberg, Martin P., *The Rise of Candidate-Centered Politics: Presidential Elections of the 1980's*. Cambridge, Mass.: Harvard University Press, 1991.

MEDIA AND CAMPAIGNS

Broh, C. Anthony, *A Horse of a Different Color*. Washington, D.C.: Joint Center for Political Studies, 1987.

Patterson, Thomas E., *The Mass Media Election: How Americans Choose Their President*. New York: Praeger, 1980.

_____ and Robert D. McClure, *The Unseeing Eye: The Myth of Television Power in Elections*. New York: Putnam, 1976.

Schramm, Martin, *The Great American Video Game: Presidential Politics in the Television Age*. New York: Morrow, 1987.

Simon, Roger, *Road Show.* New York: Farrar Strauss and Giroux, 1990.

Taylor, Paul, *See How They Run: Electing the President in an Age of Mediaocracy.* New York: Knopf, 1990.

MEDIA AND POLITICS

Alger, Dean E., *The Media and Politics*. Englewood Cliffs, N.J.: Prentice Hall, 1989.

Ansolabehere, Stephen, Roy Behr and Shanto Iyengar, *The Media Game: American Politics in the Television Age*. New York: Macmillan, 1993.

Crouse, Timothy, *The Boys on the Bus: Riding with the Campaign Press Corps*. New York: Ballantine Books, 1973.

Dye, Thomas R., Harmon Ziegler and S. Robert Lichter, *American Politics in the Media Age*. Fourth edition: Pacific Grove, Calif.: Brooks/Cole, 1992.

Entman, Robert M., *Democracy Without Citizens: Media and the Decay of American Politics*. New York: Oxford University Press, 1989.

Frantzich, Stephen E., P*olitical Parties in the Technological Age*. New York: Longman, 1989.

Graber, Doris A., ed., *Media Power in Politics*. Washington, D.C.: Congressional Quarterly, 1984.

Jamieson, Kathleen Hall, *Eloquence in an Electronic Age: The Transformation of Political Speechmaking*. New York: Oxford University Press, 1988.

Kraus, Sidney, ed., *Mass Communication and Political Information Processing*. Hillsdale, N.J.: Lawrence Erlbaum Associates, 1990.

Nimmo, Dan and James E. Combs, *Mediated Poltical Realities*. New York: Longman, 1983.

Orren, Gary R. and Nelson W. Polsby, eds., *Media and Momentum: The New Hampshire Primary and Nomination Politics*. Chatham, N.J.: Chatham House Publishers, 1987.

Ranney, Austin, *Channels of Power: The Impact of Television on American Politics*. New York: Basic Books, 1983.

Sabato, Larry J., *Feeding Frenzy: How Attack Journalism Has Transformed American Politics*. New York: The Free Press, 1991.

MEDIA AND NEWS

Blair, Gwenda, *Almost Golden: Jessica Savitch and the Selling of Television News*. New York: Avon Books, 1988.

Boyer, Peter J., *Who Killed CBS? The Undoing of America's Number One News Network*. New York: Random House, 1988.

Donaldson, Sam, *Hold On, Mr. President!* New York: Random House, 1987.

Donovan, Robert J. and Ray Scherer, *Unsilent Revolution: Television News and American Public Life, 1948-1991*. New York: Cambridge University Press, 1992.

Epstein, Edward Jay, *News From Nowhere*. New York: Vintage Books, 1973.

Friendly, Fred, *Due to Circumstances Beyond Our Control...* New York: Vintage Books, 1968.

Gans, Herbert J., *Deciding What's News: A Study of CBS Evening News, NBC Nightly News, Newsweek and Time.* New York: Pantheon, 1979.

Graber, Doris A., *Processing the News: How People Tame the Information Tide.* Second edition. New York: Longman, 1988.

Herman, Edward S., *Beyond Hypocrisy: Decoding the News in an Age of Propaganda.* Boston: South End Press, 1992.

Hewitt, Don, *Minute by Minute.* New York: Random House, 1985.

Iyengar, Shanto, *Is Anyone Responsible: How Television Frames Political Issues.* Chicago: The University of Chicago Press, 1991.

Lee, Martin A. and Norman Solomon, *Unreliable Sources: A Guide to Detecting Bias in News Media.* NY: Carol Publishing Group, 1990.

MacNeil, Robert, *The Right Place at the Right Time.* New York: Penguin Books, 1982.

Madsen, Axel, *60 Minutes: The Power and the Politics of America's Most Popular TV News Show.* New York: Dodd, Mead and Company, 1984.

Robinson, John P. and Mark R. Levy, *The Main Source: Learning from Television News.* Newbury Park, Calif.: Sage Publications, 1986.

Sanders, Marlene and Marcia Rock, *Waiting for Prime Time: The Women of Television News.* New York: Harper and Row, 1988.

Tuchman, Gaye, *Making News.* New York: The Free Press, 1978.

Whittemore, Hank, *CNN: The Inside Story.* Boston: Little, Brown and Company, 1990.

MEDIA CRITICISM

Bennett, W. Lance, *The Governing Crisis: Media, Money, and Marketing in American Elections.* New York: St. Martin's Press, 1992.

Besen, Stanley M., et. al., *Misregulating Television: Network Dominance and the FCC.* Chicago: The University of Chicago Press, 1984.

Burns, Eric, *Broadcast Blues: Dispatches From the Twenty-Year War Between a Television Reporter and His Medium.* New York: HarperCollins, 1993.

Combs, James E. and Dan Nimmo, *The New Propaganda.* New York: Longman, 1993.

Croteau, David and William Hoynes, *By Invitation Only: How the Media Limit Political Debate.* Monroe, Maine: Common Courage Press, 1994.

Dates, Jannette, L. and William Barlow, eds., *Split Image: African Americans in the Mass Media*. Washington, D.C.: Howard University Press, 1990.

Diamond, Edwin, *Good News, Bad News*. Cambridge, Mass.: The MIT Press, 1978.

_____, *Sign Off: The Last Days of Television*. Cambridge, Mass.: The MIT Press, 1982.

Fiske, John, *Media Matters: Everyday Culture and Political Change*. Minneapolis: The University of Minnesota Press, 1994.

Graber, Doris A., ed., *Media Power in Politics*. Third edition. Washington, D.C. : Congressional Quarterly Press, 1994.

Hart, Roderick, P., *Seducing America: How Television Charms the Modern Voter*. New York: Oxford University Press, 1994.

Hertsgaard, Mark, *On Bended Knee: The Press and the Reagan Presidency*. New York: Shocken Books, 1989.

Lichter, Robert S., Stanley Rothman and Linda Lichter, *The Media Elite: America's New Power Brokers*. Bethesda, Md.: Adler and Adler, 1986.

_____, Linda S. Lichter and Stanley Rothman, *Watching America: What Television Tells Us About Our Lives*. New York: Prentice Hall, 1991.

Liebling, A. J., *The Press*. New York: Pantheon, 1964.

Mankiewicz, Frank and Joel Swerdlow, *Remote Control Television and the Manipulation of American Life*. New York: Times Books, 1978.

McLuhan, Marshall and Quentin Fiore, *The Medium is the Massage*. New York: Simon and Schuster, 1967.

Metz, Robert, *CBS: Reflections in a Bloodshot Eye*. New York: New American Library, 1975.

Meyrowitz, Joshua, *No Sense of Place: The Impact of Electronic Media on Social Behavior*. New York: Oxford University Press, 1985.

Miller, Mark Crispin, *Boxed In: The Culture of TV*. Evanston, Ill.: Northwestern University Press, 1988.

Newcomb, Horace, ed., *Television: The Critical View*. Fourth edition. New York: Oxford University Press, 1987.

Postman, Neil, *Amusing Ourselves to Death: Public Discourse in the Age of Show Business*. New York: Penguin Books, 1985.

Real, Michael R., *Super Media: A Cultural Studies Approach*. Newbury Park, Calif.: Sage Publications, 1989.

Rusher, William A., *The Coming Battle for the Media: Curbing the Power of the Media Elite*. New York: Morrow, 1988.

Rushkoff, Douglas, *Media Virus: Hidden Agendas in Popular Culture*. New York: Ballantine Books, 1994.

Schwartz, Tony, *Media: The Second God*. New York: Random House, 1981.

Trotta, Liz, *Fighting For Air: In the Trenches with Television News*. New York: Simon and Schuster, 1991.

Tuchman, Gaye, ed., *The TV Establishment: Programming for Power and Profit*. Englewood Cliffs, N.J.: Prentice Hall, 1974.

Wilson, Clint C. II and Felix Gutierrez, *Minorities and Media: Diversity and the End of Mass Communication*. Newbury Park, Calif.: Sage Publications, 1986.

Winston, Brian, *Misunderstanding Media*. Cambridge, Mass.: Harvard University Press, 1986.

MASS MEDIA THEORIES

Agee, Warren K., Philip H. Ault and Edwin Emery, *Maincurrents in Mass Communication*. Second edition. New York: Harper and Row, 1989.

Klapper, Joseph T., *The Effects of Mass Media: An Analysis of Research on the Effectiveness and Limitations of Mass Media in Influencing the Opinions, Values, and Behavior of Their Audiences*. Glencoe, Ill.: The Free Press, 1960.

Severin, Werner J. with James N. Tankard, Jr., *Communication Theories: Origins, Methods, Uses*. Second edition. New York: Longman, 1988.

BOOKS BY/OR ABOUT CANDIDATES

Allen, Charles F. and Jonathan Portis, *The Comeback Kid: The Life and Career of Bill Clinton*. New York: Birch Lane Press, 1992.

Ambrose, Stephen E., *Eisenhower: Soldier General of the Army, President-Elect 1890-1952*. Volume I. New York: Simon and Schuster, 1983.

_____, *Eisenhower: The President*. Volume II. New York: Simon and Schuster, 1984.

_____, *Nixon: The Education of a Politician 1913-1962*. New York: Simon and Schuster, 1987.

Barrett, Lawrence I., *Gambling With History: Reagan in the White House*. New York: Penguin Books, 1984.

Berry, Joseph P. Jr., *John F. Kennedy and the Media: The First Television President*. Lanham, Md.: University Press of America, 1987.

Brookhiser, Richard, *The Outside Story: How Democrats and Republicans Reelected Reagan*. Garden City, N.J.: Doubleday, 1986.

Cannon, Lou, *Reagan.* New York: Putnam, 1982.

Caro, Robert A., *The Years of Lyndon Johnson: The Path to Power.* New York: Knopf, 1982.

Carter, Jimmy, *Keeping Faith: Memoirs of a President.* New York: Bantam Books, 1982.

Cohodas, Nadine, *Strom Thurmond & The Politics of Southern Change.* New York: Simon & Schuster, 1993.

Dugger, Ronnie, *The Politician: The Life and Times of Lyndon* Johnson. New York: Norton, 1982.

Ferrell, Robert H., ed., *Off the Record: The Private Papers of Harry S. Truman.* New York: Harper and Row, 1980.

_____, ed., *The Eisenhower Diaries.* Norwalk, Conn.: The Easton Press, 1989.

Ford, Gerald R., *A Time to Heal: The Autobiography of Gerald R. Ford.* New York: Harper and Row, 1979.

Goldwater, Barry M., *The Conscience of a Conservative.* Shepherdsville, Ky.: Victor Publishing Company, 1960.

_____, *With No Apologies: The Personal and Political Memoirs of U.S. Senator Barry M. Goldwater.* New York: William Morrow, 1979.

Kearns, Doris, *Lyndon Johnson and the American Dream.* New York: Harper and Row, 1976.

Kennedy, John F., *Profiles in Courage.* New York: Harper and Brothers, 1956.

Maraniss, David, *First in His Class: A Biography of Bill Clinton.* New York: Simon and Schuster, 1995.

McCullough, David, *Truman.* New York: Simon and Schuster, 1992.

Miller, Merle, *Plain Speaking: An Oral Biography of Harry S. Truman.* New York: Putnam, 1974.

Nevins, Allan, ed., *The Burden and The Glory: President John F. Kennedy, The hopes and purposes of President Kennedy's second and third years in office as revealed in his public statements and addresses.* New York: Harper and Row, 1964.

Nixon, Richard, *In the Arena: A Memoir of Victory, Defeat, and Renewal.* New York: Simon and Schuster, 1990.

_____, *The Memoirs of Richard Nixon.* Norwalk, Conn.: The Easton Press, 1988.

Noonan, Peggy, *What I Saw at the Revolution: A Political Life in the Reagan Era.* New York: Random House, 1990.

Parmet, Herbert S., *Jack: The Struggles of John F. Kennedy*. New York: Doubleday, 1980.

_____, *JFK: The Presidency of John F. Kennedy*. New York: Doubleday, 1983.

Reagan, Ronald, *An American Life*. Norwalk, Conn.: The Easton Press, 1992.

_____, *Speaking My Mind: Selected Speeches*. Norwalk, Conn: The Easton Press, 1990.

Reeves, Richard, *President Kennedy: Profile of Power*. New York: Simon and Schuster, 1993.

Renshon, Stanley A., ed., *The Clinton Presidency: Campaigning, Governing, and the Psychology of Leadership*. Boulder, Colo.: Westview Press, 1995.

Schlesinger, Arthur M. Jr., *A Thousand Days: John F. Kennedy in the White House*. Boston: Houghton Mifflin, 1965.

Sidey, Hugh, *John F. Kennedy, President*. New York: Atheneum, 1964.

Stevenson, Adlai E., *What I Think*. New York: Harper and Brothers, 1956.

Stroud, Kandy, *How Jimmy Won: The Victory Campaign From Plains to the White House*. New York: Morrow, 1977.

Truman, Margaret, *Harry S. Truman*. New York: Morrow, 1972.

Wills, Garry, *Nixon Agonistes*. Boston: Houghton Mifflin, 1970.

SPECIFIC ELECTIONS

Alpert, Eugene J., *Conventional Wisdom: A Television Viewer's Guide to the 1992 National Political Conventions*. Second edition. Washington, D.C.: C-SPAN, 1992.

Blumenthal, Sidney, *Pledging Allegiance: The Last Campaign of the Cold War*. New York: HarperCollins, 1992.

Buchanan, Bruce, *Electing A President: The Markle Commission Research on Campaign '88*. Austin, Texas: University of Texas Press, 1991.

Carlin, Diana B. and Mitchell S. McKinney, eds., *The 1992 Presidential Debates in Focus*. Westport, Conn.: Praeger, 1994.

Cook, Rhodes, *1992: Race to the Nomination: A State-by-State Guide to the Nomination Process*. Washington, D.C.: Congressional Quarterly, 1991.

Denton, Robert E. Jr., ed., *The 1992 Presidential Campaign: A Communication Perspective*. Westport, Conn.: Praeger, 1994.

Faber, Harold, *New York Times Election Handbook 1968*. Revised edition. New York: The New American Library, 1968.

Germond, Jack and Jules Witcover, *Blue Smoke and Mirrors: How Reagan Won and Why Carter Lost the Election of 1980*. New York: Viking Press, 1981.

_____, *Wake Us When It's Over: Presidential Politics of 1984*. New York: Macmillan, 1985.

_____, *Whose Broad Stripes and Bright Stars? The Trivial Pursuit of the Presidency 1988*. New York: Warner Books, 1989.

Goldman, Peter, et al., *Quest for the Presidency 1988*. New York: Simon and Schuster, 1989.

_____, *Quest for the Presidency 1992*. College Station, Texas: Texas A & M Press, 1994.

Goldstein, Michael L., *Guide to the 1988 Presidential Election*. Washington, D.C.: Congressional Quarterly, 1988.

Lichter, S. Robert, Daniel Amundson and Richard Noyes, *The Video Campaign: Network Coverage of the 1988 Primaries*. Washington, D.C.: American Enterprise Institute, 1988.

May, Ernest R. and Janet Fraser, eds., *Campaign '72: The Managers Speak*. Cambridge, Mass.: Harvard University Press, 1973.

McGinniss, Joe, *The Selling of the President 1968*. New York: Pocket Books, 1969.

Moore, Jonathan, ed., *Campaign for President: The Managers Look at '84*. Dover, Mass.: Auburn House Publishing Company, 1986.

Robinson, Michael J. and Margaret Sheehan, *Over the Wire and on TV: CBS and UPI in Campaign '80*. New York: Russell Sage Foundation, 1983.

Smith, Stephen A., ed., *Bill Clinton on Stump, State, and Stage: The Rhetorical Road to the White House*. Fayetteville, Ark.: The University of Arkansas Press, 1994.

White, Theodore H., *The Making of the President 1960: A Narrative History of American Politics in Action*. New York: Atheneum, 1961.

_____, *The Making of the President 1964*. New York: Atheneum, 1965.

_____, *The Making of the President 1968*. New York: Atheneum, 1969.

_____, *The Making of the President 1972*. New York: Atheneum, 1973.

Will, George F., *The New Season: A Spectator's Guide to the 1988 Election*. New York: Simon and Schuster, n.d.

Witcover, Jules, *Marathon: The Pursuit of the Presidency, 1972-1976*. New York: Viking Press, 1977.

SPEECHES AND RHETORIC

Andrews, James R. and David Zarefsky, *Contemporary American Voices: Significant Speeches in American History, 1945-Present.* New York: Longman, 1992.

Johannesen, Richard L., R. R. Allen and Will A. Linkugel, *Contemporary American Speeches.* Sixth edition. Dubuque, Iowa: Kendall/Hunt, 1988.

Lott, Davis Newton, *The Presidents Speak: The Inaugural Addresses of the American Presidents,* From Washington to Clinton. New York: Henry Holt and Company, 1994.

Ryan Halford Ross, *American Rhetoric from Roosevelt to Reagan: A Collection of Speeches and Critical Essays.* Prospect Heights, Ill.: Waveland Press, 1983.

Windt, Theodore, *Presidential Rhetoric: 1961 to the Present.* Third edition. Dubuque, Iowa: Kendall/Hunt, 1983.

THE POLITICAL PROCESS

Ailes, Roger with Jon Kraushar, *You Are The Message: Secrets of the Master Communicators.* Homewood, Ill.: Dow Jones-Irwin, 1988.

Alexander, Herbert with Anthony Corrado, *Financing the 1992 Election.* Armonk, N.Y.: M.E. Sharpe, 1995.

_____, with Monica Bauer, *Financing the 1988 Election.* Boulder, Colo.: Westview Press, 1991.

_____, with Brian A. Haggerty, *Financing the 1984 Election.* Lexington, Mass.: Lexington Books, 1987.

_____, *Financing the 1980 Election.* Lexington, Mass., D. C: Heath, 1983.

_____, *Financing Politics: Money, Elections, and Political Reform.* Washington, D.C.: Congressional Quarterly Press, 1976.

_____, *Financing the 1972 Election.* Lexington, Mass.: Heath, Lexington Books, 1976.

_____, *Financing the 1968 Election.* Lexington, Mass.: D.C. Heath, 1971.

_____, *Financing the 1964 Election.* Princeton, N.J.: Citizens' Research Foundation, 1962.

Bailey, Thomas A., *Presidential Saints and Sinners.* New York: The Free Press, 1981.

Bartels, Larry M., *Presidential Primaries and the Dynamics of Choice.* Princeton, N.J.: Princeton University Press, 1988.

Beasley, Maurine H., *Eleanor Roosevelt and the Media: A Public Quest for Self-Fulfillment.* Urbana, Ill.: University of Illinois Press, 1987.

Brownstein, Donald, *The Power and the Glitter: The Hollywood-Washington Connection.* New York: Pantheon, 1990.

Edwards, George C. III with Alec M. Gallup, *Presidential Approval: A Sourcebook.* Baltimore, Md.: The Johns Hopkins University Press, 1990.

Frantzich, Stephen E. and Stephen L. Percy, *American Government: The Political Game.* Dubuque, Iowa: Brown and Benchmark, 1994.

Heard, Alexander, *The Costs of Democracy.* Chapel Hill, N.C.: The University of North Carolina Press, 1960.

Jamieson, Kathleen Hall, *Dirty Politics: Deception, Distraction, and Democracy.* New York: Oxford University Press, 1992.

Lutz, William, *Double-Speak: From "Revenue Enhancement" to "Terminal Living"—How Government, Business, Advertisers, and Others Use Language to Deceive You.* New York: Harper Perennial, 1989.

Matalin, Mary and James Carville, *All's Fair: Love, War, and Running for President.* New York: Random House, 1994.

Moore, David M., *The Super Pollsters: How They Measure Public Opinion in America.* New York: Four Walls Eight Windows, 1992.

Parry, Robert, *Fooling America: How Washington Insiders Twist the Truth and Manufacture the Conventional Wisdom.* New York: Morrow, 1992.

Phillips, Kevin, *Arrogant Capitol: Washington, Wall Street, and the Frustration of American Politics.* Boston: Little, Brown and Company, 1994.

_____, *Post-Conservative America: People, Politics, and Ideology in a Time of Crisis.* New York: Vintage Books, 1982.

_____, *The Emerging Republican Majority.* Garden City, N.J.: Doubleday, 1969.

_____, *The Politics of the Rich and Poor: Wealth and the American Electorate in the Reagan Aftermath.* New York: Random House, 1990.

Piven, Frances Fox and Richard A. Cloward, *Why Americans Don't Vote. Updated edition.* New York: Pantheon, 1989.

Polsby, Nelson W. and Aaron Wildavsky, *Presidential Elections: Contemporary Strategies of American Electoral Politics.* Eighth edition. New York: The Free Press, 1991.

Romney, Ronna and Beppie Harrison, *Momentum: Women in American Politics Now.* New York: Cross Publishing Company, 1988.

Sabato, Larry J., ed., *Campaigns and Elections: A Reader in Modern American Politics.* Glenview, Ill.: Scott, Foresman and Company, 1989.
_____, *PAC Power: Inside the World of Political Action Committees.* New York: Norton, 1990.
Smith, Hedrick, *The Power Game: How Washington Works.* New York: Random House, 1988.
Stockman, David A., *The Triumph of Politics: The Inside Story of The Reagan Revolution.* New York: Avon Books, 1987.
Teachout, Terry, ed., *Beyond the Boom: New Voices on American Life, Culture, and Politics.* New York: Poseidon Press, 1990.
Thomas, Cal, *The Things That Matter Most.* New York: HarperCollins, 1994.
Wolfinger, Raymond E. and Steven J. Rosenstone, *Who Votes?* New Haven, Conn.: Yale University Press, 1980.

BOOKS OF TIME PERIODS

Gitlin, Todd, *The Sixties: Years of Hope, Days of Rage.* New York: Bantam Books, 1987.
Goodwin, Doris Kearns, *The Fitzgeralds and the Kennedys: An American Saga.* New York: Simon and Schuster, 1987.

Halberstam, David, *The Fifties.* New York: Villard Books, 1993.
Hughes, Emmet John, *The Ordeal of Power: A Political Memoir of the Eisenhower Years.* New York: Atheneum, 1963.
Manchester, William, *The Glory and the Dream: A Narrative History of America 1932-1972.* New York: Bantam Books, 1974.
Will, George F., *The Leveling Wind: Politics, the Culture, and Other News,* 1990-1994. New York: Viking Press, 1994.

NEW TECHNOLOGY ISSUES

Bianculli, David, *Teleliteracy: Taking Television Seriously.* New York: Continuum, 1992.
Dizard, Wilson P. Jr., *The Coming Information Age: An Overview of Technology, Economics, and Politics.* Third edition. New York: Longman, 1989.
Howard, Herbert H., Michael S. Klievman and Barbara A. Moore, *Radio, TV, and Cable Programming.* Second edition. Ames, Iowa: Iowa State University, 1994.
Lamb, Brian et. al., *C-SPAN: America's Town Hall.* Washington, D.C.: Acropolis

Books, 1988.

Maney, Kevin, *Megamedia Shakeout: The Inside Story of the Leaders and Losers in the Exploding Communications Industry.* New York: John Wiley and Sons, 1995.

Pavlik, John V. and Everette E. Dennis, *Demystifying Media Technology.* Mountain View, Calif.: Mayfield Publishing, 1993.

TEXTS FOR SCHOOLS AND COLLEGES

The books that would be more appropriate for students and/or teachers of elementary school are designated with an (E); those for secondary school with an (S); and those for college with a (C). A number of other books listed in other categories within this bibliography could be used in schools and colleges where appropriate.

Bloomquist, David, *Elections and the Mass Media.* Washington, D.C.: The American Political Science Association, 1982. (C)

Considine, David M. and Gail E. Haley, *Visual Messages: Integrating Imagery into Instruction.* Englewood, Colorado: Teacher Ideas Press, 1992. (E,S,C)

Frantzich, Stephen, *Using C-SPAN in the Classroom: A Faculty Guide to Integrating Public Affairs Programming.* West Lafayette, Ind.: Purdue Research Foundation, 1989. (C)

Hanson, Jarice and Alison Alexander, eds., *Taking Sides: Clashing Views on Controversial Issues in Mass Media and Society.* Guildford, Conn.: The Dushkin Publishing Group, 1991. (C)

Jamieson, Kathleen Hall and Karlyn Kohrs Campbell, *The Interplay of Influence: Mass Media and Their Publics in the News, Advertising, Politics.* Belmont, Calif.: Wadsworth Publishing Company, 1992. (C)

Jeffries, Leo W., *Mass Media Processes.* Second edition. Prospect Heights, Ill.: Waveland Press, 1994. (C)

Lusted, David, *The Media Studies Book: A Guide for Teachers.* New York: Rutledge, 1991. (E,S,C)

O'Reilly, Kevin and John Splaine, *Critical Viewing: Stimulant to Critical Thinking.* Pacific Grove, Calif.: Critical Thinking Press and Software, 1987. Updated and Revised, 1996. (S)

Shaver, James P., ed., *Handbook of Research on Social Studies Teaching and Learning.* New York: Macmillian Publishing Company, 1991. (E,S,C)

Splaine, John and Pam Splaine, *Educating the Consumer of Television: An Interactive Approach.* Pacific Grove, Calif.: Critical Thinking Press and Software, 1992. (E, S)

DATE DUE

FEB 2 0 2000	